The Fasciae

ANATOMY, DYSFUNCTION AND TREATMENT

Serge Paoletti

ILLUSTRATIONS BY PETER SOMMERFELD

EASTLAND PRESS • SEATTLE

Originally published in French as *Les Fascias: Rôle des Tissus dans la mécanique humaine*
by Sully Editions in 1998, and a second edition in 2002

English edition ©2006 by Serge Paoletti

Published by Eastland Press, Inc.
P.O. Box 99749
Seattle, WA 98139, USA
www.eastlandpress.com

Library of Congress Control Number: 2006920183
International Standard Book Number. 978-0-939616-53-4
Printed in China

2   4   6   8   10   9   7   5   3

Translated by Antiope Traductions
Cover design by Patricia O'Connor
Cover Illustration by Peter Sommerfeld

Book design by Gary Niemeier

Table of Contents

Preface

The APONEUROSES, LIGAMENTS, RETINACULA, and the elastic laminae of arteries, among many, many other structures, are all part of the fascial system and, by extension, part of the connective tissues. If one goes back still further to embryology, these all relate to the mesenchyma. All soft tissues, and in particular the fasciae, derive originally from the same embryonic layer, the mesoderm, which is actually at the origin of all bodily tissues apart from the skin and the mucosae. The mesoderm gives rise not only to those elements conventionally defined as fasciae, but also to cartilage and bone, which in reality are no more than particularly dense forms of fascial tissue.

The fasciae constitute an uninterrupted sheet of tissue that extends from the head to the feet and from the exterior to the interior. This is a perfectly continuous system that is suspended from bony structures to form a fully integrated supporting framework.

The ubiquitous fasciae not only invest the external surface of all the body's diverse structures— muscles, organs, nerves, vessels—but also form the internal matrices which support these structures and maintain their integrity. For this reason we can say that the fasciae constitute an envelope responsible for maintaining structure and anatomical form throughout the body, right down to the level of the individual cells, which are bathed in the ground substance of the fascial system. This superficial envelope over the entire body is repeatedly divided to create an ever-more complex network of compartments and connections. For enhanced efficacy, the fasciae are anchored to the skeleton, not by simple contiguity, but rather by insinuation into the osseous trabeculae via Sharpey's fibers.

In all the diverse anatomical sites of the body, the fasciae show remarkable adaptability in terms of their shape, structure and composition. The fascial elements in muscular tissues, conventionally described as tendons and ligaments, are the densest and therefore the strongest tissues, making them suitable for the job that they are required to perform – anchoring muscle and bone to bone. Conversely, the areolar tissue, which makes up the fasciae that invest the glands, is relatively loosely structured.

Distributed throughout the body, the fasciae play a fundamental role in human physiology. This role takes many forms: maintaining posture; maintaining the structure of the organs; guaranteeing the anatomic integrity of diverse internal structures; and investing the muscles to support them and allow them to generate force. One important role of the fascial system is to provide "transmission belts" for the endogenous and exogenous forces which the body generates itself and to which it is subjected from the outside. This function allows the body to move in an efficient, coordinated manner and respond to external phenomena. However, these same networks of fascial elements can also participate in the propagation of pathological forces, thereby mediating a chain reaction of damaging consequences. One of their key functions is the absorption of shocks.

Finally, these tissues play a primary role in many physiological transport processes and defense mechanisms. The ground substance of the fasciae is in direct contact with the cells of the body and provides a medium of exchange that ensures efficient communication between the extracellular and intracellular environments. The fasciae constitute the first defensive barrier against external insults and come into play prior to any kind of mobilization of the immune system. The fasciae are thus capable of autonomous decision-making. One could even speak of this system as a "peripheral brain."

The fasciae are endowed with "cellular memory" derived from embryonic growth, which is manifested in the form of a regular, rhythmic motility. This "cellular memory" enables the fasciae to register any deformation which they undergo and, up to a certain point, to correct it. However, if the deformation is too extreme, it is beyond correction by the fasciae acting alone and progressive pathology can result.

Our hands can sense that motility as well as the evidence of damage to the tissues. With certain specific techniques and manipulations, we can help the fasciae to resolve nonphysiological stress patterns and thereby regain their normal functionality.

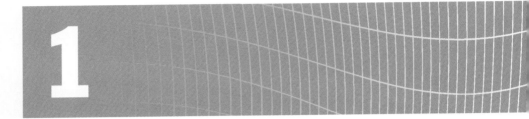

Embryology

ANY UNDERSTANDING OF functional anatomy must start at the source. For this reason we begin with a brief review of human embryology starting at the beginning of the second week, when the different layers first appear in the zygote, and continuing through the end of the eighth week, when embryogenesis is complete. The subsequent stages of the process correspond to fetal development.

Formation of the Two-layered Embryonic Disk

During the second week, the blastocyst which was formed during the first week becomes solidly embedded in the mucosal lining of the uterus via the trophoblast.

The embryoblast and trophoblast subsequently develop to form different kinds of tissue.

The trophoblast differentiates to form:

- the syncytiotrophoblast
- the cytotrophoblast

The embryoblast gives rise to the two layers of the embryonic disk:

- the epiblast (ectoderm)
- the hypoblast (endoderm)

Initially, the epiblastic cells are connected to the cytotrophoblast, but later, small fissures appear between the two layers of cells. These fissures soon become confluent and give rise to the amniotic cavity. A junction—the amnioembryonic junction—is established between the amnioblast and the epiblastic layer.

The trophoblast then develops rapidly, particularly at the embryonic pole where intracytoplasmic vacuoles appear. These later become the lacunar spaces.

During this time, away from the embryonic pole, flattened cells peel off the internal surface of the cytotrophoblast to form the exocoelomic (Heuser's) membrane, which is continuous with the edge of the hypoblast; together, they form the exocoelomic cavity, which soon becomes the primary or primitive yolk sac (Fig. 1-1).

Fig. 1-1 Twelve-day Blastocyst

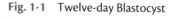

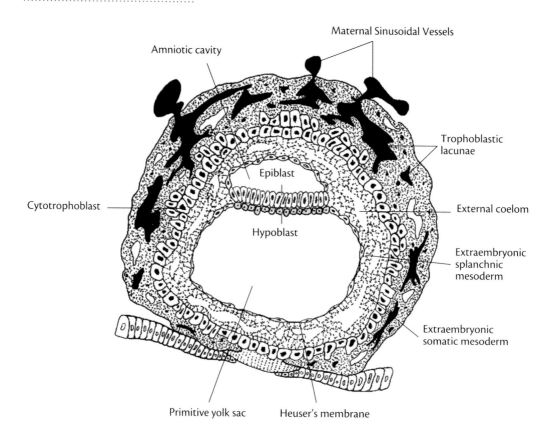

After eleven to twelve days of development, the blastocyst represents a small bump on the lining of the uterus. At the same time, syncytial cells penetrate more deeply into the stroma, secreting a substance that dilates the maternal capillaries so that they turn into larger-caliber sinusoidal vessels.

The lacunary syncytium is now continuous with the endothelial cells of the vessels and maternal blood passes into the lacunary system. Finally, arterial and venous capillaries in the lacunary spaces become patent. Maternal blood circulates through the trophoblastic lacunary system as a result of the difference in pressure between the arterial and venous capillaries. This constitutes the beginning of uteroplacental circulation.

Cells continue to peel off at the internal surface of the cytotrophoblast to form the extraembryonic mesoderm. Soon, large cavities appear in these tissues giving rise to a new cavity, the extraembryonic coelom, that is going to surround the primitive yolk sac and the amniotic cavity (except where it joins the trophoblast).

The extraembryonic mesoderm lining the cytotrophoblast and the amnion is called the extraembryonic somatopleure. The layer lining the yolk sac is called the extraembryonic splanchnopleure.

Around day thirteen, the layer of embryonic ectoderm that started to develop into epithelial cells at the internal surface of the exocoelomic membrane continues to proliferate and forms a new cavity, the secondary yolk sac, which is also known simply as the yolk sac (Fig. 1-2). This is much smaller than the exocoelomic cavity; significant fragments of the latter are eliminated, although occasionally exocoelomic cysts persist in the external coelom.

Fig. 1-2   Thirteen-day Blastocyst

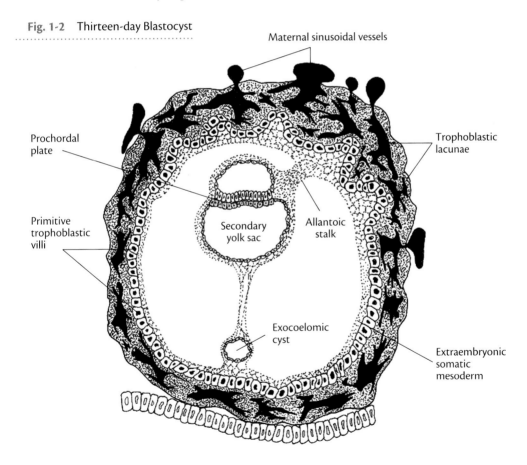

Maternal sinusoidal vessels

Prochordal plate

Trophoblastic lacunae

Primitive trophoblastic villi

Secondary yolk sac

Allantoic stalk

Exocoelomic cyst

Extraembryonic somatic mesoderm

Toward the end of the second week, the embryonic disk consists of two superimposed layers of tissue:

- the epiblastic layer, forming the floor of the amniotic cavity, and
- the hypoblastic layer, forming the roof of the secondary yolk sac

Formation of the Three-layered Embryonic Disk

The third week of development is characterized by the appearance of the primitive streak on the ectodermal surface opposite the amniotic cavity (Fig. 1-3). It is at this point that the embryo can be said to have a craniocaudal axis as well as dorsal and ventral surfaces and left and right sides. The slightly raised mass of cells at the cranial end of the primitive streak is called the primitive node, the primitive knot, or Hensen's knot.

Fig. 1-3 Embryonic Disk at the End of Week 2

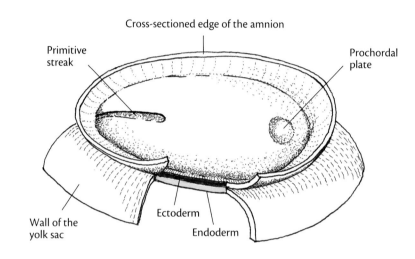

Cross-sectioned edge of the amnion

Primitive streak

Prochordal plate

Wall of the yolk sac

Ectoderm

Endoderm

To mark the effect of the primitive streak, the epiblastic layer will hereafter be referred to as ectoderm and the hypoblastic layer as endoderm. Some cells from the deep ectodermal layer migrate out over the surface of the disk in the direction of the primitive streak, and then turn downwards into the furrow to create an invagination. The then continue their migration in a lateral direction between the ectodermal and endodermal layers to give rise to the intraembryonic mesoderm. This process is called gastrulation.

The cells which form the invagination in the region of the primitive node migrate further in a cranial direction as far as the prochordan plate where they form another invagination, which has the same shape as the finger of a glove. This invagination which originates at the primitive node is called the notochordal (archenteric) canal (Fig. 1-4). Advance of the notochordal canal is blocked in the prochordan region by the close association between the ectoderm and the endoderm.

Around day seventeen, the chordomesoderm separates the ectoderm and endoderm completely, except around the cloacal membrane and the prochordan plate; the notochordal canal closes, giving rise to a dense chord, the definitive notochord. The primitive streak regresses around week four (Fig. 1-5).

On about day twenty, the embryo is attached to the trophoblast by only the allantoic stalk, which will later give rise to the umbilical chord.

Fig. 1-4 Dorsal View of Cell Migration over Embryonic Disk

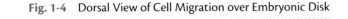

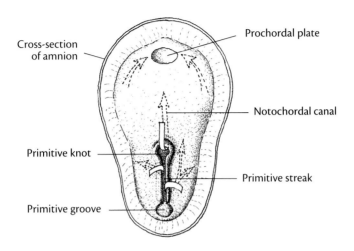

Fig. 1-5 A. Cephalocaudal Cross-section through a Seventeen-day Embryo
B. Section through the Embryonic Cranium
C. Section in the Area of the Primitive Streak

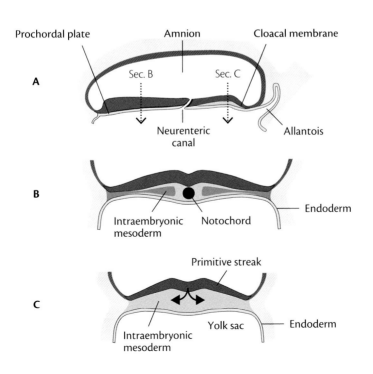

Sheet Differentiation and Embryonic Development

Between weeks four and eight, the three different sheets each give rise to a variety of specific tissues and organs (Fig. 1-6). During this period, the appearance of the embryo completely changes and, by the end of month two, the major external features of the body are easily recognizable.

Fig. 1-6 Embryonic Cross-sections of Liver, Spleen, & Stomach

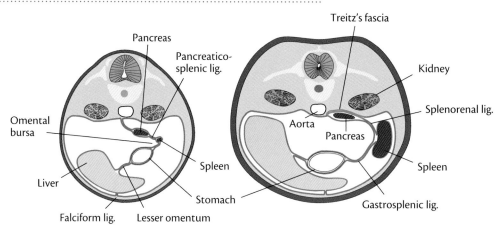

DERIVATIVES OF THE MESODERM

Towards day seventeen, mesodermal cells on either side of the mid-line proliferate and form the paraxial mesoderm. The lateral mesoderm remains thin and is referred to as the lateral plate; it later splits to form two distinct layers (Fig. 1-7):

Fig. 1-7 Cross-sections Showing Mesodermal Development

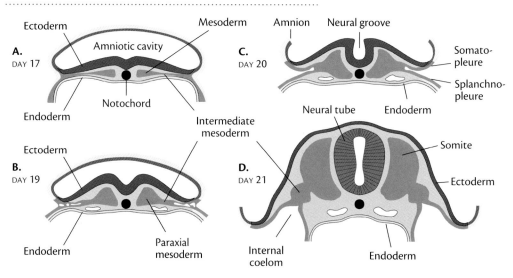

- one will form the amnion, the intraembryonic somatopleure, also known as the somatic or parietal mesoderm layer;
- the other will form the yolk sac, the intraembryonic splanchnopleure, also known as the splanchnic or visceral mesoderm layer

Together, these two layers define the edges of the coelom. The tissue between the paraxial mesoderm and the lateral plate is called the intermediate mesoderm.

Paraxial mesoderm

Towards the end of week three, the paraxial mesoderm condenses to form the somites, which develop as forty-two to forty-four pairs arranged along the craniocaudal axis.

At the beginning of week four, the somites begin migrating towards the notochord to form the sclerotomes. These consist of immature connective tissue cells with an enormous capacity for differentiation; they can differentiate to form cells as diverse as:

- fibroblasts, which form various types of fibers: reticular fibers, collagen fibers, elastic fibers;
- chondroblasts, which synthesize cartilage;
- osteoclasts, which synthesize bone

After migration of the sclerotome, the somite wall becomes the dermomyotome. From the inner side of this derives the myotome, which will give rise to muscles in the corresponding segment. After detachment of the myotome, the remaining cells spread out under the ectodermal layer, which will later grow out over them and form the dermis and subcutaneous tissues.

Intermediate mesoderm

These cells give rise to both the urinary and genital systems and are sometimes known as the nephrotome. In the cervical and upper thoracic regions, this tissue gives rise to a very primitive set of kidneys known as the pronephroi. While these soon degenerate, they do set up a system of ducts that run caudally and open into the cloaca, which are used by later iterations of the kidneys. In the caudal region, these cells give rise to the nephrogenic cord, which will form the kidney when that organ's secretory system has developed (Fig. 1-8).

Lateral plate

As described above, the lateral mesoderm differentiates to form the somatopleure and splanchnopleure, which line the intraembryonic coelom.

When the embryo folds back on itself (Fig. 1-9):

- the somatopleure forms, with the ectoderm covering it and the lateral and ventral walls of the embryo;

Fig. 1-8 Cross-section through the Intermediate Mesoderm: Day 21

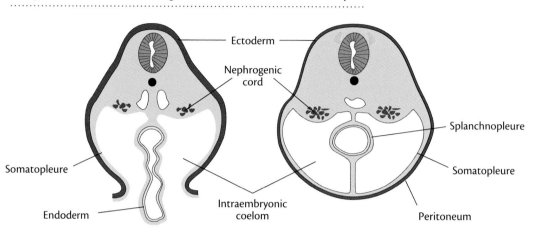

Ectoderm

Nephrogenic cord

Splanchnopleure

Somatopleure

Somatopleure

Endoderm

Intraembryonic coelom

Peritoneum

Fig. 1-9 Cross-sections at Days 24, 26, & 28 Showing Embryonic Involution

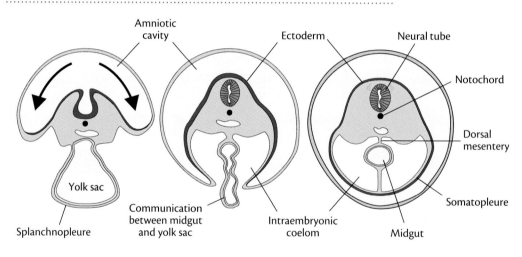

Amniotic cavity

Ectoderm

Neural tube

Notochord

Dorsal mesentery

Yolk sac

Communication between midgut and yolk sac

Intraembryonic coelom

Somatopleure

Splanchnopleure

Midgut

- the splanchnopleure will coil around the endoderm to form the wall of the digestive tube

Around the middle of week three, mesodermal cells on each side of the median line and opposite the prochordan plate will begin to form the primordium of the future heart and blood vessels. The extraembryonic vessels form projections which fuse with the walls of the intraembryonic vessels to establish communication between the embryonic and placental circulatory systems.

The mesoderm then gives rise to different derivatives:

- connective tissues, cartilage, bone, and both striated and smooth muscle
- the pericardium, the pleura, and the peritoneum
- blood and lymphoid cells
- the walls of the heart, the blood vessels, and the lymphatics

- the kidneys, the gonads, and their respective excretory and secretory systems
- the cortex and medulla of the suprarenal glands
- the spleen

Therefore, the connective tissues—the principal subject of this text—belong to the mesoderm and, more specifically, to the mesenchyma.

Mesenchymal cells proliferate and migrate to all regions of the embryo, filling in otherwise unoccupied spaces and intercalating between the cells which make up the organs. All the constituents of connective tissue derive directly or indirectly from this primitive system. Mesenchymal cells are the precursors for most cell types found in adult connective tissue. Certain cells do not further differentiate and multiply in an immature form. These undifferentiated cells play a central role in the processes of growth and repair as well as in certain defense mechanisms. Such immature or stem cells retain their embryonic potential for proliferation and can later differentiate to generate new lineages of more specialized cell types.

The mesoderm, as explained above, is covered by two layers of tissue: an external layer, the ectoderm, one part of which will cover the mesoderm during embryonic development; and an internal layer, the endoderm, that will be supported by the mesoderm.

DERIVATIVES OF THE ECTODERM

At the beginning of week three, at the same time that the notochord is being formed, the nascent central nervous system begins to develop in the form of a thickened plate of ectoderm—the neural plate—which expands toward the primitive streak.

The lateral edges of this plate subsequently rise to form the neural crests, and a median depression becomes the neural groove. The neural crests later gradually approach one another, eventually forming the neural tube (Fig. 1-10).

Therefore, the early nervous system consists of a straight cylindrical portion, the medullary chord, and a larger cephalic part, the primary brain vesicles, which, towards the end of week four, give rise to the auditory and optic vesicles.

When the embryo folds back on itself, the ectoderm splits into two different parts. One part will be enveloped by the mesoderm and will form the nervous system, sending out multiple processes during development into the mesoderm and then into the endoderm. The other part will go on to cover the mesoderm and form the epidermis.

The ectoderm therefore gives rise to the following systems and structures:

- the central and peripheral nervous systems
- the sensory epithelia and sense organs
- the epidermis and its appendages (hair, nails, and cutaneous glands)
- the pituitary gland
- the enamel of the teeth

Fig. 1-10   Development of Neural Crest, Neural Groove and Neural Tube

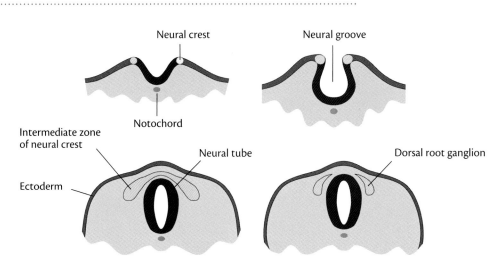

DERIVATIVES OF THE ENDODERM

Due to the growth of the central nervous system and of the somites, the embryo undergoes folding in the longitudinal and transverse planes. This results in the enclosure of part of the yolk sac in the resultant cavity. This internalization of part of the yolk sac paves the way for the eventual formation of the digestive tube (Fig. 1-11).

The endoderm will give rise to the anterior, middle, and inferior segments of the intestine (Fig. 1-12):

- the anterior intestine will be provisionally closed by the closing (pharyngeal) membrane

Fig. 1-11   Cross-section through the Duodenum

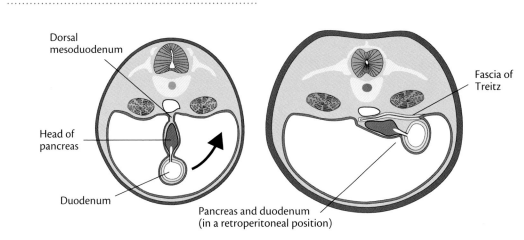

Fig. 1-12 Sagittal section of Endoderm development

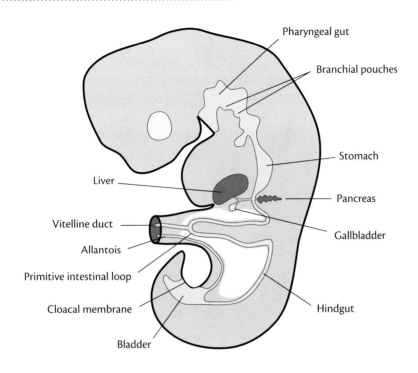

- Pharyngeal gut
- Branchial pouches
- Stomach
- Liver
- Pancreas
- Vitelline duct
- Gallbladder
- Allantois
- Primitive intestinal loop
- Cloacal membrane
- Hindgut
- Bladder

- the posterior intestine will be closed by the cloacal membrane that subsequently splits to form the genitourinary and anal membranes (Fig. 1-13)

At this point, due to folding in the lateral plane, compartmentalization of the embryo begins with the formation of the abdominal wall defining a tubular cavity, which will eventually become the intestine.

Due to the formation of the caudal fold at the end of week four, the umbilical vesicle and the allantoic stalk fuse to give rise to the umbilical cord.

Fig. 1-13 Different Developmental Stages of the Cloacal Membrane

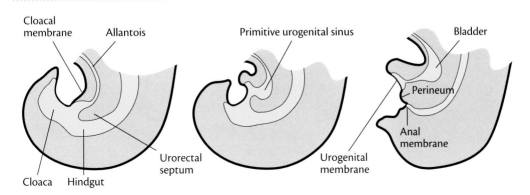

Cloacal membrane
Allantois
Primitive urogenital sinus
Bladder
Perineum
Anal membrane
Urorectal septum
Urogenital membrane
Cloaca
Hindgut

The endoderm therefore gives rise to the following structures:

- the epithelial linings of the digestive tube, the bladder, and the urethra
- the epithelial lining of the airways
- the epithelial linings of the tympanic cavity and the auditory tubes
- the parenchyma of the tonsils, the thyroid, parathyroid, and thymus
- the esophagus, stomach, liver, gallbladder, pancreas, and intestine
- the broncotracheal system
- the closing membrane, the cloaca, and the allantois
- the branchial clefts

Between weeks five and eight, all these systems will continue developing and various embryonic structures will begin to become apparent, including the primordia of the limbs, the organs (in their correct location), and the head.

This is a period of organization during which the fetus is formed. The next stage focuses on the growth of already established structures.

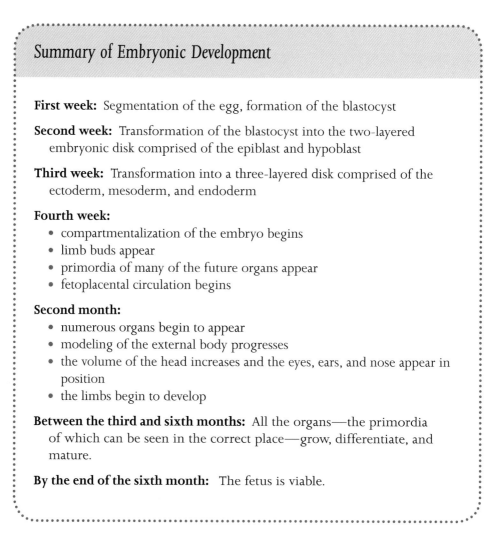

Summary of Embryonic Development

First week: Segmentation of the egg, formation of the blastocyst

Second week: Transformation of the blastocyst into the two-layered embryonic disk comprised of the epiblast and hypoblast

Third week: Transformation into a three-layered disk comprised of the ectoderm, mesoderm, and endoderm

Fourth week:
- compartmentalization of the embryo begins
- limb buds appear
- primordia of many of the future organs appear
- fetoplacental circulation begins

Second month:
- numerous organs begin to appear
- modeling of the external body progresses
- the volume of the head increases and the eyes, ears, and nose appear in position
- the limbs begin to develop

Between the third and sixth months: All the organs—the primordia of which can be seen in the correct place—grow, differentiate, and mature.

By the end of the sixth month: The fetus is viable.

DERIVATIVES OF THE VARIOUS LAYERS

Mesoderm

- connective tissue, cartilage, bone, and both striated and smooth muscle
- pericardium, pleura and peritoneum
- blood and lymphoid cells
- walls of the heart, blood vessels, and lymphatics
- kidneys, gonads, and their respective excretory and secretory systems
- cortex and medulla of the suprarenal glands
- spleen
- muscular linings and the connective tissues of the digestive system
- epithelial linings of the digestive tube, bladder, and urethra

Endoderm

- epithelial lining of the airways
- epithelial linings of the tympanic cavity and auditory tubes
- parenchyma of the tonsils, thyroid, and parathyroid
- thymus
- esophagus, stomach, liver, gallbladder, and bile ducts
- pancreas and intestine
- tracheobronchial system
- allantois and the inner layer of the cloacal and closing membranes

Ectoderm

- central and peripheral nervous systems
- sensory epithelium and sense organs
- epidermis and appendages (hair, nails, cutaneous glands)
- mammary glands
- pituitary gland
- tooth enamel

Built of three superimposed layers, the embryo grows and develops in a continuous sequence. Growth is accompanied by compartmentalization of the embryo: vertical compartmentalization with the appearance of the cephalocaudal curvature, and lateral compartmentalization with the development of the walls and cavities. During this process the various organs of the body are positioned (Fig. 1-14 & 1-15). As part of the same process the buds of the upper and lower limbs appear.

As of the moment when the ovum first encounters the spermatozoon, the fertilized egg is in continual, lively movement, movement which terminates in the formation of an organism of extraordinary complexity.

Each of the layers is continually combining, associating, and interacting with its neighbors to grow and develop into the different parts of the human body, all this with an amazing degree of consistency and organization. Cells from a single primordial tissue can differentiate to form bones, muscles, fasciae, nerves, skin, the liver, or the spleen—and all this in a near-perfect process, since errors are relatively rare.

Fig. 1-14   Section through an Embryo at the Beginning of Week 4

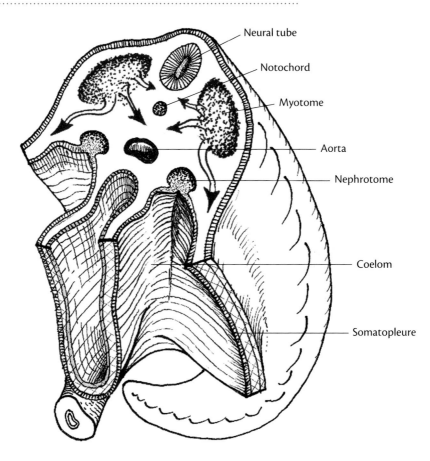

This growth all occurs according to a pulse—the natural rhythm of the developing organism.

By the end of the second month, as we have seen, the fetus is in place. The subsequent stages are concerned primarily with growth and maturation. However, the rhythm of life which was triggered at fertilization will not now cease until death. It is this rhythm that paces the growth, movement, and performance of all the functions of the human body. The same rhythm derived from embryological memory can be found in the cranium, the fasciae, the organs, everywhere: the rhythm with which the body adapts to the potentially devastating perturbations of the external world, maintaining a stable, constant internal milieu, and thereby maintaining its equilibrium and health.

With our hands, we can sense this rhythm and determine whether the body or any part of it is in harmony or is dysfunctional.

Fig. 1-15   Section through an Embryo at the End of Week 4

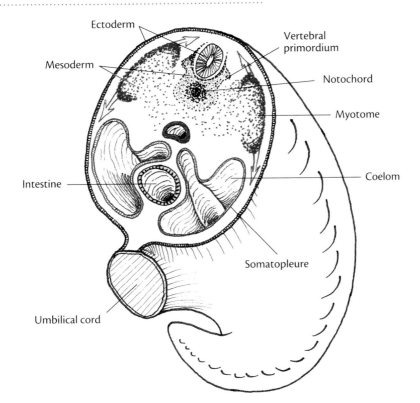

The Mechanisms Underlying Embryonic Development

How does an egg give rise to a human being? How is such a degree of complexity generated during development?

Embryonic development involves cytochemical, biochemical, biokinetic, and biodynamic phenomena, all of which play a part in directing and organizing the growing cells and tissues.

HISTOLOGICAL AND BIOCHEMICAL PHENOMENA

"Cells know where they are in the embryo on the basis of the local concentrations of specific morphogens."   —C. Nusslein-Volhard

Studies performed with *Drosophila* have led to the identification of these morphogens. Some thirty genes in *Drosophila* define the 'manager' of the embryo. Only three of them encode molecular signals that determine structure along the anteroposterior axis. Each of these three signaling proteins appears in only one specific site and triggers the creation of a gradient based on one specific morphogen.

One signal is active in the anterior part that will give rise to the head and thorax. A second signal is active in the abdomen, and a third determines the structures situated at the two ends of the larva.

A concentration gradient of the Bicoid protein is established in the very earliest stages with the highest concentration found at the anterior end. A certain critical threshold concentration is required for this signaling molecule to exert any effect. Once this threshold is reached, a specific gene is transcribed into messenger RNA, which is subsequently translated to form a protein. A concentration gradient of the protein acts on two or three genes determining only two or three regions of activation.

The Bicoid messenger RNA contains all the information necessary for a cell to recognize, transport, and bind it. Furthermore, it always moves in the same direction along structural elements called microtubules.

The Nanos protein is active in the posterior part. Gradients of both the Bicoid and Nanos proteins can only become established if there are no cellular membranes to block their diffusion. However, in most animals, cellular membranes separate the different regions of the egg from the very earliest stages of development. The dorsoventral axis of the *Drosophila* embryo is determined by a gradient that is established across cellular membranes. Similar types of gradient are probably important in other organisms.

The Dorsal protein determines the first embryonic structures along the dorsal-vertebral axis. This protein acts as both an activator and an inhibitor of transcription in the nucleus of the cell: when its concentration exceeds a given threshold, it activates a pair of genes, whereas when its concentration is below that threshold, it acts as an inhibitor of another pair of genes.

Therefore, when different concentrations of the Dorsal protein in different nuclei define a gradient, each of the pairs of genes is expressed differently on either one side or the other of the embryo.

The concentration of the Dorsal protein is uniform in the embryo; it is its intracellular distribution that varies along the dorsoventral axis. A protein called Cactus binds to the Dorsal protein to block its entry into the nucleus. However, at the ventral surface of the embryo, more than ten other proteins interact to release the Dorsal protein from the Cactus protein.

The proteins are activated by a signal. Molecular relay systems based on several different proteins transmit information about the gradients between the different compartments. Finally, even if a protein is uniformly distributed at the beginning, its transport into the nucleus can cause activation by generating a concentration gradient.

All the activation pathways studied to date lead to the formation of a morphogen gradient that ultimately controls the rate of transcription; depending on its concentration, the gradient activates or inhibits the transcription of one or more target genes. Synergistic interactions between different factors, or between several copies of the same factor, can regulate the rate of transcription of specific genes.

Certain morphogen gradients exert only one effect and only when the morphogen concentration is above a critical threshold; if the threshold is not reached, the target gene is not activated. In other cases, the response depends on the absolute concentration of the morphogen; this type of gradient is key when it comes to generating complexity.

Interactions between different factors which influence transcription can hugely modify the responses to gradients. This helps explain how combinations of basically simple systems can give rise to highly complex structures.

The superimposition of several different gradients in a given region of the embryo increases the resolution of such systems and therefore provides another mechanism for generating complexity.

Combinatorial regulation and the exploitation of concentration gradients mean that a limited number of genes can give rise to a vast repertory of different developmental mechanisms. In the case of *Drosophila*, the gradients trigger the expression of genes in transverse bands. These bands correspond to regions of the egg that will eventually become the different segments of the larva. Within the areas corresponding to these macroscopic bands, other systems generate yet finer bands that directly determine the characteristics of each segment of the embryo. When the egg divides and forms individual cells, the transcription factors can no longer diffuse. At later stages, when the 'manager' of the embryo is established, signals transmitted between neighboring cells play the predominant role.

Embryologists have found that these results not only apply to *Drosophila*, but to the animal kingdom as a whole, leading to the hope that one day we will better understand the development of the human embryo.

BIOKINETIC AND BIODYNAMIC PHENOMENA

The kinetic development of the embryo has been studied by Blechschmidt, who defined the important role played by metabolic fields, of which there are eight:

Corrosion fields

A corrosion field is established when two layers of epithelial cells associate to form a thin, two-layered membrane. The cells in contact undergo necrosis and disappear, permitting communication between the fluids or with overlying tissues. This type of field is established from the second week on and is found between the mesonephric tubules and the nephrotic canal, and in developing blood vessels. The two dorsal aortas enter into contact and their median membrane degenerates to form a single vessel. There are many other examples of corrosion fields, for example, the bucconasal, buccopharyngeal, cloacal, and seminiferous membranes.

Densation fields

Densation fields are important in skeletal development. This type of field is composed of packed spherical cells which are associated with very limited amounts of interstitial substance. The exact amount of interstitial substance distinguishes dense fields from sparse ones.

Primoridal cellular masses, from which an organ is formed, are called blastemas. For example, cartilaginous tissue derives from blastema, but only a part of the blastema itself becomes cartilage. This is also the origin of ligaments and capsules.

Normal organic development is initiated not from inside the cell, but from outside. Densation fields are characterized not only by the general position of the filed, but by specific positions of cells and their nuclei. Following Blechshmidt and Gasser (1978), let us use the development of the trachea as an example.

Example: tracheal development. The dorsal epithelium is thicker than the ventral. The cells adjacent to the epithelium are elongated and aligned tangentially; they will give rise to the tracheal muscles and the fibrous membrane. On the ventral side, the stroma corresponds to a densation field with an aggregate of many spherical cells in a limited amount of interstitial substance.

The dorsal epithelium grows more rapidly than the ventral, which brings about lengthening of the cells and induces their tangential alignment. Compression at the ventral level causes the cells to become spherical. These cells proliferate, condense, and become cartilaginous tissue (Fig. 1-16).

Fig. 1-16   Densation Fields

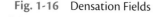

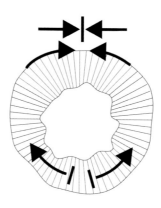

The biokinetic principle of densation fields also applies to the development of other structural formations such as the ribs, which are subject to high pressure as a result of the increasing mass of the heart and liver. Densation fields also influence the development of the nasal septum and many other structures.

Differentiation in a densation field arises from a biomechanical phenomenon resulting from a biodynamic process. The cells in the fields have no specific orientation, that is, they are submitted to the same tension in all directions and consequently become spherical.

Contusion fields

In a densation field spherical cells flatten out and are transformed into cartilage cells. When this process occurs on a circular plane along the longitudinal axis of densation and proceeds from the center toward the periphery, the result is called a contusion field. Contusion fields are always surrounded by perichondrium that fuses with loose peripheral mesenchyma.

A densation field is a zone of condensation of round cells, while a contusion field is a zone of compression where cells flatten out.

Contusion fields are especially relevant in skeletal development. The limb buds are surrounded by a membrane at the interior of which cells proliferate in all directions, creating equivalent forces at all points and pushing the intercellular fluid toward the periphery. This creates the conditions necessary for a contusion field.

Contusion fields thus develop within densation fields when there is resistance along the longitudinal axis due to the growth of spherical cells. Resistance to growth brings about compression that, in turn, tends to flatten out the cells and transform them into cartilage-forming cells.

Distusion fields

The term *distusion* is used to refer to a process where there is an outward pressure along longitudinal axes against a spring-like resistance. These fields are also relevant to the development of the skeletal system. In the limbs of a two-month embryo, the old cartilage is localized in the proximal portion and the more recent cartilage in the distal portion. Furthermore, the cartilage-forming cells appear first in the central portion, that is, far from the vascular peripheral mesenchyma. If we take the example of a phalange under compression, the cells lose their fluid and are not near any blood supply. The shape of the cells changes and they become spherical. They grow primarily along a single axis. This type of growth is due to the occurrence of a tumefaction that is referred to as a distusion field.

The pattern of growth and tumefaction parallels the longitudinal axis of the pre-existing cartilage. Such cartilage grows as if it were being acted upon by a piston. The compression is so great that fluid is squeezed out, a capsule forms around the cells, and the process of calcification begins.

Retention fields

Retention fields represent an aggregation of internal tissue cells that began by being undifferentiated and which grow slowly in a direction dictated by a stretching motion that originates with neighboring tissues. The stretching forces to which these growing cells are subject gradually transform them into fibrous connective tissue that gives rise to tendons, ligaments, and aponeuroses.

The forces created by a retention field cause peripheral parts to grow more rapidly, a key factor in the determination of human morphology.

Dilatation fields

Dilatation fields occur when tissues are stretched longitudinally without transverse compression; this leads to a thinning of the tissues. These fields are relevant to the development of the muscular system. The development of this system differs from site to site, but the fundamental principles are the same for all muscles.

The primordium of cardiac muscle is under less pressure from the coelomic fluid outside than from the blood inside, with the result that it tends to dilate. This dilatation will gradually bring about a reaction in the form of contraction. The result of this process of dilatation and contraction is that cardiac cells are able to move about relatively freely with respect to one another. The heart steadily dilates and this increases the resistance of the circular muscle fibers. The volume then increases, but, since it is fixed at either end, the organ as a whole develops in an oval shape.

Dilatation fields are also important in the development of the skeletal muscular system. The rapidly expanding somites on the periphery of the dermatome grow out in the cranial and caudal directions, following the general direction of growth in the embryo.

As a result, the cells under the dermatome align themselves on a craniocaudal axis parallel to the axis of the neural tube. The muscle cells become thinner in the dilatation field and, at the same time, intracellular myofibrils begin to form. The transverse striations are poorly defined at first.

After the first month, a line of nuclei becomes distinct as a result of the growth of the muscle cells. Once the cells of the dermatome have aligned along the ectodermal membrane, the myotome cells orient at right angles to the septum.

Dilatation fields are usually involved in the development of the curvature of stretched muscle cells as well as in the development of tendons. Dilatation fields are thus characteristic not only of longitudinal growth but also of transverse expansion.

The muscular primordium in densely packed areas cannot dilate in the transverse direction. Therefore, in such areas, it undergoes compression which leads to the formation of tendinous tissue. In these regions, the fluid content of the interstitial substance is very low, making it extremely viscous.

Tendons, like all highly compressed tissues, have a restrictive function. Other types of tissue with only minimal elasticity, and which serve to contain or restrict other structures, are the fasciae and the intermuscular septa.

Dilatation fields in embryonic cartilaginous tissue are essential for the growth of muscles and tendons. The growth of cartilage parallels muscular growth. All muscles have passive functions before becoming capable of active contraction. The more rapidly muscle cells grow, the more richly they become innervated and the sooner they can contract.

Dilatation fields also are important in the development of the intestinal tract.

Parathelial loosening fields

Loosening fields are created by congestion of the interstitial substance in the internal tissues where cellular catabolites exert a major effect. When the quantity of catabolites increases, the volume of the interstitial substance increases in parallel and vesicles tend to fuse together.

At the beginning of development, loose fields within the mesoderm are precursors for the formation of the blood vessels and lymphatics. One particular group, the parathelial loose fields, is important in the development of glandular structures.

Detraction fields

Detraction fields are involved in the development of bones. From the topological point of view, there are three types of bone tissue:

- membranal bones that develop from stretched connective tissue
- cartalaginous bones that develop from cartilage
- bones that develop from already existing bone tissue

The kinetics of development of all three types show that their development is characterized by the fact that it is always accompanied by expansion of the intercellular substance in response to some kind of force.

Extracellular processes are primordial for the triggering of the ossification process.

Mesenchyma cells sliding along a rigid support become compressed. The fluid is squeezed out of the interstitial substance, which hardens as a consequence. These regions in which cellular aggregates slide and become compressed against some hard, supporting structure are called detraction fields

By way of example, take the development of a frontal bone. The primordium of the dura mater is a layer of connective tissue which is under tension. Strong pulling by the orbital septum in the direction of the lower face causes the membrane to separate into two laminae, and a center of ossification becomes established on the external layer. It is the primordium of the external layer which is responsible for the tension. The internal layer accommodates the expansion of the growing arachnoidea mater. Its intercellular fluid is squeezed out and, as a result, the interstitial substance hardens and a point of condensation for the development of bone tissue is created.

Once hardened, the internal part of the tissue in the area of condensation loses its potential for growth. The tissue forms a coating around the center of condensation and then spreads by cellular proliferation. Over time, the centers of ossification advance as divergent lines, radiating from the points of condensation (detraction fields).

Anatomy of the Fasciae

TO OUR KNOWLEDGE, there is no text of anatomy that deals specifically with the fasciae. This is why we have decided to present an outline of this subject here. This chapter represents the result of a review of many different treatises and articles. We do not pretend to have succeeded in concentrating all the many and various aspects of the anatomy of the fasciae into a few pages—indeed, we have tried to avoid presenting too much detail. However, it appeared to us essential to present in one chapter an overview of how these tissues are organized at the macroscopic level, as well as some idea of their anatomy and histology at the microscopic level. This background information is important when it comes to understanding their various roles and mechanisms of action. Nonetheless, for readers who may be less than enthralled by a long rehash of anatomical details, or who are interested in only a simple survey of fascial anatomy, succinct summaries are presented at the end of each section together with tables wthich recap how each fascial element relates to its corresponding structures.

Superficial Fascia

The superficial fascia lies between the adipose layer of the dermis and subcutaneous cellular tissue. The true superficial fascia starts at the zygomatic arch, inserts into the maxilla, and terminates at the ankles and wrists.

It is absent:

- on the face
- over the upper part of the sternocleidomastoid muscle
- at the nape of the neck
- over the sternum

• at the buttocks

This tissue layer serves as the point of origin for lymphatic vessels, and also plays a key role in cellular nutrition and respiration. The degree of severity of burns is evaluated on the basis of the damage suffered by the superficial fascia.

External Fasciae

EPICRANIAL APONEUROSIS

The epicranial aponeurosis (also known as the galea aponeurotica) is an extensive, fibrous lamina that covers the entire convex surface of the skull like a skullcap. It is separated from the periosteum by loose cellular tissue which allows the layers to slide over one another to some extent. Conversely, it is tightly attached to the skin so these layers are obliged to move together.

In the anteroposterior direction, the epicranial aponeurosis joins the occipital and frontal muscles. It is inserted posteriorly, on the external occipital protuberance as well as on the superior nuchal line. Its lateral extension corresponds to the temporal and masseteric aponeuroses, and it terminates on the supramastoid ridge, the external auditory tube, and the subcutaneous tissue of the masseteric region.

Temporal fascia

Thick and very strong, the temporal fascia extends from the superior temporal curved line and the space included between the two curved lines to the zygomatic bone as two laminae that attach to the lips of the arch; from there it extends as the masseteric fascia (*Fig. 2-1; Table 2-1*).

Table 2-1   Connections of the epicranial aponeurosis

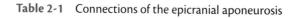

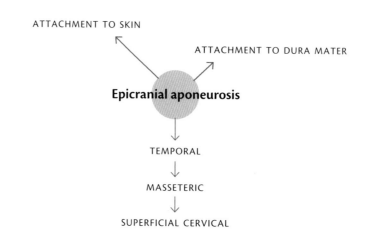

Fig. 2-1 Lateral Fasciae of the Face

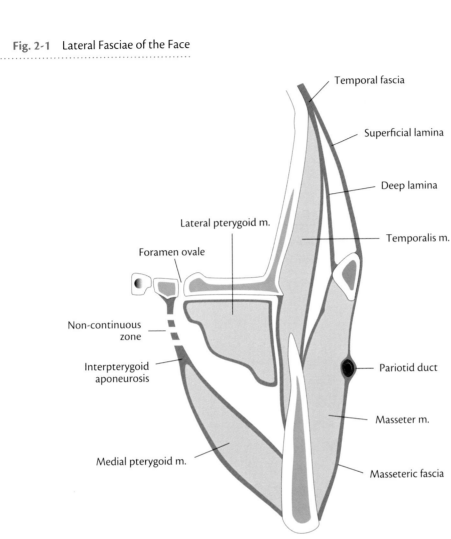

Temporal fascia

Superficial lamina

Deep lamina

Lateral pterygoid m.

Temporalis m.

Foramen ovale

Non-continuous zone

Interpterygoid aponeurosis

Pariotid duct

Masseter m.

Medial pterygoid m.

Masseteric fascia

Masseteric fascia

It is inserted:

- behind, on the posterior rim of the ascending ramus of the mandible
- in front, skirting the masseter muscle and then passing over its posterior surface before inserting on the anterior edge of the ascending ramus
- above, attaching to the zygomatic arch
- below, attaching to the lower edge of the maxillary where it is continuous with the superficial cervical fascia
- in the back, along the posterior edge where it joins the parotid fascia and splits to invest the parotid duct

Fasciae of the face

The fasciae of the face (Fig. 2-2) consist of:

- A superficial fascial sheet, itself composed of two different layers, namely a thin superficial layer and a stronger deep layer. These two layers invest the muscles which control facial mobility and link them to the deep fascia.
- A deep fascial sheet which is thicker and inelastic. This is separated from the superficial fascia by loose areolar connective tissue. The deep fascia invests the bones, the cartilage, the jaw muscles, and various visceral structures. Like the superficial fascia, it constitutes a continuous sheath that resembles and is derived from the temporal and parotid-masseteric fasciae. The deep fascia supports the deep vessels and the nerves innervating the jaw.

Fig. 2-2   Fasciae of the Face

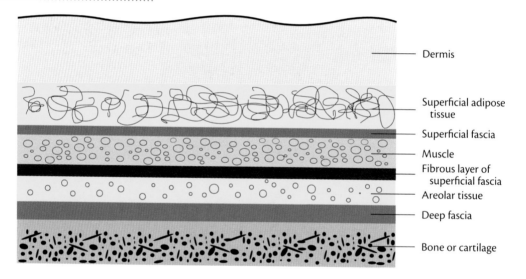

- Dermis
- Superficial adipose tissue
- Superficial fascia
- Muscle
- Fibrous layer of superficial fascia
- Areolar tissue
- Deep fascia
- Bone or cartilage

SUPERFICIAL CERVICAL FASCIA

This fascia (Fig. 2-3) forms a sealed sheath in the neck. It is attached, at the top:

- to the superior nuchal line
- to the mastoid process
- to the cartilage of the external auditory tube
- to the masseteric aponeurosis and the lower edge of the jaw

It is thus an extension of the epicranial aponeurosis.
   At the bottom:

- on the anterior edge of the jugular notch of the sternum
- on the anterior face of the manubrium of the sternum
- on the upper face of the clavicle
- on the posterior edge of the spine of the scapula

A fibrous extension emanates from its deep surface along the anterior edge of the trapezius muscle. This deep extension is joined inside to the aponeuroses of the scalene muscles.

Its anterior part, where it is covered by the muscles of the skin, is thin relative to the rest of it.

The superficial cervical fascia splits to provide a sheath for the sternocleidomastoid and trapezius muscles. It runs in front of the hyoid bone onto which it inserts. Laterally it expands, forming a sheath within which the digastric muscle slides and folds back upon itself.

Fig. 2-3   Superficial and Middle Cervical Fasciae

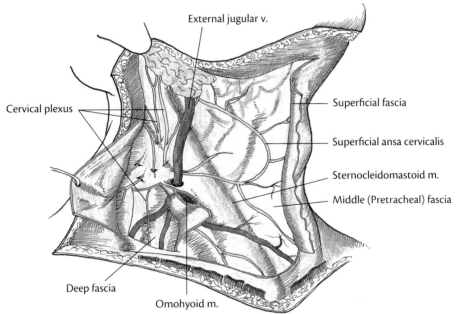

It joins with the middle cervical fascia in the anterior, superior, and median sub-hyoid regions.

In their lower regions, the two fascial sheets separate to insert on the sternal notch, one in the anterior edge, the other in the posterior edge. The sternal space thus defined is sealed on the outside by adhesion of the middle fascia to the anterior edge of the sheath of the sternocleidomastoid muscle in front, and the aponeurosis of the trapezius muscle behind.

Below the hyoid bone, this fascia splits to form the aponeurosis of the sub-maxillary glands. Behind, it invests the parotid gland and, together with the masseteric aponeurosis, constitutes its sheath.

Lateral to the anterior edge of the sternocleidomastoid muscle, a small band detaches and inserts at the angle of the mandible. This small maxillary ligament supports and stretches the sternocleidomastoid aponeurosis so that the muscle remains flat and protects the underlying bundle of vessels and nerves (including the carotid vessels, the internal jugular vein, and the vagus nerve).

Behind, on the median line, the superficial cervical fascia presents a fibrous fold extending from the external occipital protuberance to the sixth cervical vertebra and, occasionally, as far as the first thoracic vertebra. This is the posterior cervical ligament, the median part of which is attached to the spinous processes of the vertebrae.

The posterior cervical ligament is a very strong sheet of tissue which is attached to aponeurotic extensions of the trapezius, splenius, and rhomboid muscles, and the serratus posterior superior. In some people, this structure is in the form of a cord the size of a pencil which juts out when the head is inclined.

The superficial cervical fascia splits several times to invest all the muscles of the nape of the neck. The anterior jugular veins initially cross the surface of this fascia in sheaths derived from the basal sheet. Subsequently, they pass through the fascia.

On the surface of the superficial cervical fascia lie the superficial branches of the cervical plexus: C2, C3, C4. It should be noted that all these, as well as the external jugular vein, pass through the fascia at the posterior edge of the sternocleidomastoid muscle.

The superficial cervical fascia is continuous with the fasciae of the trunk and the lower limbs as well as those of the upper limbs.

FASCIAE OF THE TRUNK

The fasciae of the trunk are continuous with the superficial cervical fascia. At the top, they are inserted into:

- the sternum
- the clavicle
- the scapular spine

From there, the fascial system extends out in two directions to form the fasciae of the trunk on the one hand, and those of the upper limbs on the other hand. There are numerous divisions all along the way forming intermuscular septa and sheaths for the numerous muscles in these parts of the body.

The fasciae of the trunk invest the sacrolumbar mass of the sacrospinal muscle and the pectoral, trapezius, and latissimus dorsi muscles. Emanations from this complex form the aponeuroses of the deep muscles, including the quadratus lumborum, the external intercostal muscles, and the muscles associated with the vertebral column.

Aponeuroses originating in the abdomen are those of the internal and external oblique muscles, the transversus abdominis, and the rectus abdominis (Fig. 2-4).

Posterior Fasciae

Two different fascial elements will be distinguished: a thoracolumbar system with a median portion which is especially well defined where it inserts into the spinous processes of the vertebrae; and a lower part which constitutes the

Fig. 2-4   Cross-section through the Abdomen

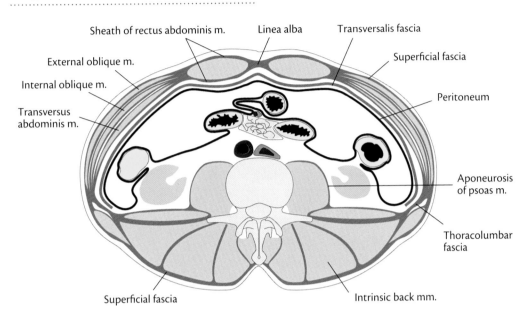

Sheath of rectus abdominis m.   Linea alba   Transversalis fascia

External oblique m.

Superficial fascia

Internal oblique m.

Transversus
abdominis m.

Peritoneum

Aponeurosis
of psoas m.

Thoracolumbar
fascia

Superficial fascia   Intrinsic back mm.

lumbar fascia, a very strong sheet which is inserted into the spinous processes of the vertebrae, the sacrum, and the iliac crest. The latter extends down into the gluteal aponeurosis and then into the lower limbs; it extends on the sides to form the fasciae of the external and internal oblique muscles of the abdomen.

The posterolateral part of the fascia is reinforced by the aponeurosis of the latissimus dorsi, which links the pelvis and the upper limb since it terminates at the intertubercular sulcus. Along the way, it sends out an extension that attaches to the lower angle of the scapula.

The superior part of the iliocostal fascia is reinforced by the aponeurosis of the trapezius muscle to which it is attached.

The lumbar fascia is attached along the median line to the spinous processes of the vertebrae, particularly those of L2 to S2. This very strong structure is made of interwoven oblique, transverse, and vertical fibers, indicating that this region is subject to extreme forces. The lumbar fascia becomes progressively thicker and gives off numerous strong ligaments, including those of the sacrum and the sacrospinal and sacrotuberous ligaments.

Anterior Fascia

The upper part of the anterior fascia is derived from the aponeuroses of the subclavius muscle and the pectoralis major and minor. In the median part of the fascia, where there are no muscles, it is attached to the sternum.

This complex is continuous on its sides with the aponeuroses of the deltoids and the axillary fascia. It is indirectly continuous with the aponeurosis of the latissimus dorsi muscle and joins with the posterior fasciae and those of the upper limbs (Fig. 2-5).

Fig. 2-5 Thoraco-abdominal Fasciae

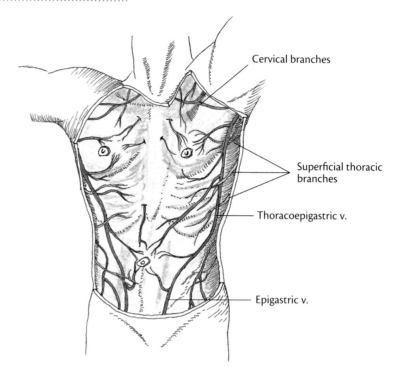

Cervical branches

Superficial thoracic branches

Thoracoepigastric v.

Epigastric v.

Continuity in the lower medial and lateral regions is formed by the aponeuroses of the oblique and transverse muscles of the abdomen, and the sheath investing the rectus muscle.

All these aponeuroses meet on the median line, creating the linea alba, where the differently aligned fibers of the two meet. The actual contact is relatively loose.

The fascial tissue above the umbilicus is always looser than that below it; this explains why most linea alba hernias are supra-umbilical. However, the looseness is functional during pregnancy: when the swollen uterus migrates upward through the abdominal cavity, the linea alba moves out of the way and thus permits dilatation of the abdomen without any concomitant generation of excess pressure which could lead to the compression of the underlying organs. The same phenomenon occurs in people who put on weight: accumulation of fat around the omentum leads to displacement of the fibers of the linea alba.

The linea alba inserts superiorly into the xiphoid process and inferiorly into the pubic symphysis where it continues into the suspensor ligament of either the penis or the clitoris.

It should be noted that the anterolateral part of the abdomen is the only place in the body where there is no rigid structure. This is the reason why the abdominal fasciae divide and dive deep into the body. With the aponeurosis of the transverse muscle, they eventually penetrate down as far as the internal abdominal surface where they come into direct contact with the fascia transversalis and the peritoneum.

Also to be noted in speaking of the abdomen is the presence of the internal and external inguinal rings, which represent weak points where intestinal loops can become externalized, causing hernia. The inguinal canal contains the round ligament in the female and the spermatic cord in the male. When the testis descends into the scrotum during adolescence, it travels the canal and creates, in the wake of its passage, an invagination:

- in the peritoneum constituting the tunica vaginalis
- in the fascia transversalis constituting the fibrous tunica
- in the bundles of the small oblique and transverse muscles that will constitute the tunica muscularis or the cremaster muscle

The latissimus dorsi and trapezius muscles stretch the posterior aponeurosis, and the pectoralis major acts on the anterior aponeurosis.

The posterior part of the sheath of the rectus abdominis is interrupted about three centimeters below the umbilicus to form a strong, semi-circular line called the arcuate line of the sheath of the rectus abdominis muscle. This is easy to palpate in many subjects and should not be confused with the root of the mesentery, which is much deeper down.

The aponeuroses of the abdominal muscles join with the lower part of the abdomen in a line that extends from one anterior superior iliac spine to the other, across the entire width of the pubic symphysis.

Several groups of fibers come together to form the inguinal ligament, including one set of fibers derived from the fascia lata. Thus, the canal acts as a relay center and represents a point of continuity between the fascial systems of the abdomen and the lower extremities. Other fibers originate in the iliac fascia and the transversalis fascia, so the inguinal ligament also represents a point at which the abdominal wall meets the internal surface of the abdomen.

Reinforcements of the supra-pubic abdominal fasciae (Fig. 2-6) correspond to the reflex inguinal ligament (Colle's ligament), the lacunar ligament (Gimbernat's ligament), and the interfoveolar ligament (Hesselbach's ligament).

Iliac Fascia

The iliac fascia, an offshoot of the superficial abdominal fascia, warrants special attention for two reasons: First, by virtue of its situation, it invests the psoas muscle which, apart from the longus colli muscle of the neck, is the only muscle which is inserted in the anterior vertebrae and which therefore passes inside a body cavity. Second, by virtue of its numerous relationships with other structures like the kidneys, the ureter, and the descending and ascending colon.

Moreover, it is the iliac fascia which splits to invest the lumbar plexus. It also spans the entire width of the internal iliac fossa, reaching from the superior insertion point of the psoas muscle as far as its insertion into the trochanter, from where it continues as the fascia lata femoralis.

The upper part of the iliac fascia is thin but gradually thickens as it descends down into the pelvis. It contains the tendon of the psoas minor muscle (when extant).

Fig. 2-6   Vertical and anteroposterior sections of the inguino-abdominal and inguinocrural regions

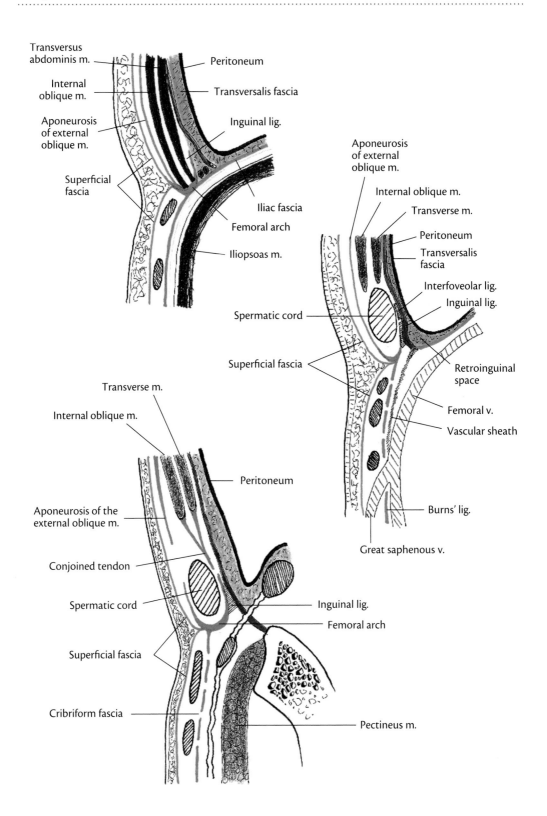

The iliac fascia inserts:

On the inside

- into the lumbar vertebrae where it forms passages for the lumbar arteries and veins
- at the base of the sacrum
- at the superior opening of the pelvis where it invests the external iliac artery and vein, keeping these vessels in place on the medial edge of the psoas muscle

On the outside

- into the aponeurosis of the quadratus lumborum muscle and along the external edge of the psoas
- into the iliolumbar ligament
- into the internal lip of the iliac crest

At the top

It thickens to create the arcuate ligaments at the top of the psoas, into which the corresponding part of the diaphragm inserts (another example of fascial continuity).

At the bottom

The iliac fascia is strongly attached to the external half of the inguinal ligament (again, a relay center and point of continuity with the abdominal fascia). Its internal surface forms the iliopectineal arch and then continues as far as its insertion into the trochanter, where it is continuous with the fascia lata.

This description shows that the iliac fascia joins the lumbar column and the internal iliac fossa to form an osteofibrous compartment, the abdominal part of which is completely closed. This compartment is open on the side of the thigh above the lateral part of the inguinal ligament.

The iliac fascia is basically composed of bundles of fascial tissue, running in a transverse direction, to which are joined a few vertically oriented bundles. A sheet of cells separates the iliac fascia from the peritoneum. The iliac fascia invests the psoas muscle without being attached to it—the two are separated by a cellular serous membrane. The nerves of the lumbar plexus are intimately bound to this fascia.

Summary of the Fasciae of the Trunk

This fascial system is continuous with the superficial cervical fascia at the scapular girdle. It terminates below at the upper periphery of the pelvis, where it is continued by the fasciae of the lower limb.

The anterior and posterior median insertion points for this fascial system are:

- the sternum
- the spinous processes of the vertebrae

The fasciae are divided to invest the various muscles present in the abdomen and the thorax.

Superiorly the fascial sheet is continuous with the axillary aponeuroses and the fascial elements of the upper limb.

In the lower trunk, where there are very few muscles, the fasciae become very strong. They give rise to many laminae emanating in different directions to support the structures in the thorax and abdomen.

In the abdomen, the fascia splits repeatedly and penetrates deeply, eventually joining with the transversalis fascia.

The deepest posterior split constitutes the iliac fascia.

At the level of the pelvis, the fasciae of the trunk are continuous with the perineal fasciae, particularly the superficial and middle perineal fasciae.

Finally, at the anterior level, via the umbilical ligament, the fasciae of the trunk are connected to the deep perineal fascia and the fasciae associated with the organs of the lesser pelvis.

UPPER LIMB FASCIAE

This fascial system joins the superficial cervical fascia at the clavicle, the acromion, and the process of the scapula. It is also continuous with the fasciae of the greater pectoral and latissimus dorsi muscles, and the axillary fascia.

Although it is only of medium thickness throughout, it is nevertheless stronger on the side of the extensor muscles than on that of the flexors. A complex network of nerves and lymphatics runs through the tissue. In the bottom third of the forearm, the fascia is pierced by the cutaneous branch of the radial nerve (Fig. 2-7).

It is pierced at the level of the fold of the elbow by the lateral antebrachial cutaneous nerve. In the lower third of the arm, there is the opening for the basilic vein (to which it is attached) and from which emerge the anterior and ulnar branches of the medial antebrachial cutaneous nerve. Its superior lateral part contains the accessory of the medial antebrachial cutaneous nerve into which there is an anastomosis of the intercostal arteries.

The cephalic vein runs along the external edge of the upper limb. At the level of the fold of the elbow, it is regularly linked to the basilic vein via the median cubital vein, and travels part of the way in association with the lateral cutaneous antebrachial nerve. It ascends in the deltopectoral sulcus where it passes through the deltoid and clavipectoral aponeuroses before emptying into the axillary vein.

Fig. 2-7   Upper Limb Fasciae

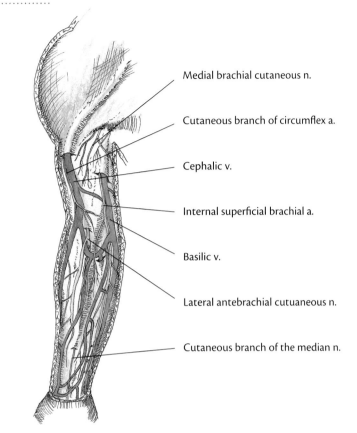

— Medial brachial cutaneous n.

— Cutaneous branch of circumflex a.

— Cephalic v.

— Internal superficial brachial a.

— Basilic v.

— Lateral antebrachial cutuaneous n.

— Cutaneous branch of the median n.

Numerous intermuscular septa derive from the inner surface of the fascia of the upper limb; repeated splitting of these sheets results in the creation of sheaths for all the different muscles of the limb.

There are points of attachment at the elbow and at the wrist where it is continuous with the palmar aponeurosis.

Each successive portion of the upper limb will be considered separately in the following order: the shoulder, the arm, the forearm, and the hand.

Shoulder Fasciae

The fascia of the shoulder is continuous with the superficial cervical fascia. Its lateral anterior and posterior portions correspond to the aponeurosis of the pectoralis major muscle. In front, it is composed of the aponeurosis of the deltoid muscle, and behind, those of the infraspinous and supraspinous muscles (Fig. 2-8).

The fascia is split behind the pectoralis major by the axillary clavipectoral fascia and the subclavian aponeurosis, which is reinforced by the medial coricoclavicular (conoid) ligament. From the lower edge of the subclavian aponeurosis, a membrane detaches, which is attached to the pectoralis minor muscle. This structure splits into two separate sheets:

- an anterior sheet, which joins with the aponeurosis of the pectoralis major underneath, and is attached to the skin at the base of the axilla

Fig. 2-8 Axilla: Vertical, Anteroposterior Cross-section

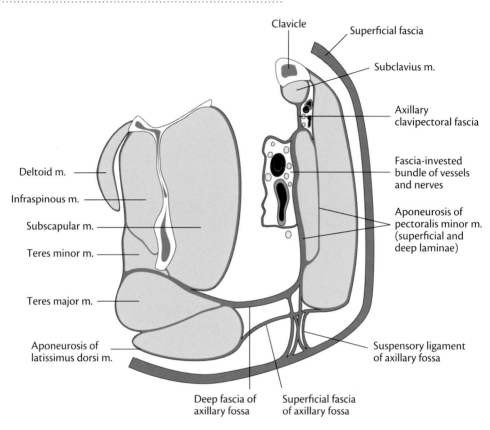

Clavicle

Superficial fascia

Subclavius m.

Axillary clavipectoral fascia

Fascia-invested bundle of vessels and nerves

Aponeurosis of pectoralis minor m. (superficial and deep laminae)

Deltoid m.

Infraspinous m.

Subscapular m.

Teres minor m.

Teres major m.

Aponeurosis of latissimus dorsi m.

Suspensory ligament of axillary fossa

Deep fascia of axillary fossa

Superficial fascia of axillary fossa

- a posterior sheet, which continues into the deep axillary aponeurosis and also attaches to the skin of the armpit via the clavipectoral fascia

The inferior medial part of the fascia of the shoulder constitutes the aponeurosis of the base of the axillary cavity and is composed of two fascial membranes, namely, the superficial and the deep fasciae:

Superficial fascia

The superficial lamina extends from the inferior edge of the pectoralis major to the inferior edges of the latissimus dorsi and the teres major muscles.

Deep fascia

The deep fascia is a four-sided sheet which is joined in the front to the deep layer of the suspensory ligament. From that point of attachment, it passes back to attach itself to the entire length of the axillary edge of the scapula. Outside, the deep fascia adheres to the anterior face of the tendon of the long biceps muscle. Its posterior part comes into contact with the latissimus dorsi and teres major muscles.

Its inferior medial edge joins the aponeurosis of the serratus superior muscle.

Outside, it is joined to the coracobrachial aponeuroses of the coracobrachialis and the biceps. Behind, it constitutes the axillary arch, which invests a bundle of vessels and nerves.

Brachial Fascia

The brachial fascia is continuous with the fasciae of the shoulder. It terminates at the elbow where it inserts into the oleocranon and the medial and lateral epicondyles of the humerus. An extension of the tendon of the biceps—a genuine aponeurotic tensor—is attached to its anterior part (Fig. 2-9).

Fig. 2-9 Upper Arm: Horizontal Cross-section at the Two-thirds Distal Point

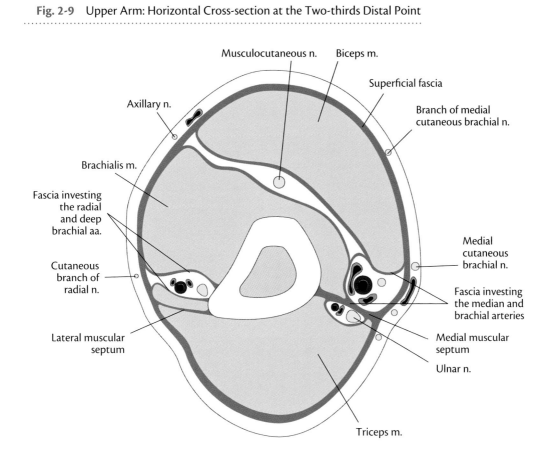

It forms two septa, which are oriented in the sagittal plane:

- the lateral intermuscular septum
- the medial intermuscular septum

In the sagittal plane, these septa secure the aponeurosis to the bone and permit the various groups of muscles to operate with maximum efficiency, with the septa as their strong point.

Lateral intermuscular septum

The lateral intermuscular septum of the arm originates in the intertubercular sulcus and unites with the posterior edge of the tendon of the deltoid muscle. It inserts along the whole length of the external edge of the humerus as far as the epicondyle. It separates and provides insertion points for both the anterior and posterior muscles. It is crossed at an oblique angle by the radial nerve and the deep brachial artery.

Medial intermuscular septum

The medial intermuscular septum is wider and thicker than its lateral homologue, originating at the posterior edge of the intertubercular sulcus. It continues into the tendon of the coracobrachial muscle with which it unites and, to a certain extent, insinuates itself. It is inserted along the entire length of the humerus as far as the medial epicondyle of the humerus. It sends out a thin, fibrous extension, the medial brachial ligament, which extends from the superior end of the medial intermuscular septum to the lesser tubercle of the humerus, passing behind the coracobrachial muscle.

This ligament separates the triceps muscle from the anterior brachial muscle and provides both of them with insertion points.

The anterior ulnar nerve crosses the septum in its middle and remains associated with its posterior part.

Sheaths for various muscles emanate from the deep surface of this fascia, namely, the biceps, coracobrachial, anterior brachial, and triceps muscles. An aponeurotic sheet at its superior part separates the long portion of the triceps from the rest of the muscle. The inferior part of this sheet is continuous with the sulcus of the radial nerve and houses both the nerve and the deep brachial artery in its own aponeurosis.

Between the biceps and the anterior brachial muscles lies a thin fascial layer, which separates them and contributes to their mobility. This sheet is continuous with the antebrachial fascia.

In the interior part, in contact with the interior intermuscular septum, runs the brachial canal, which contains the brachial artery and vein, and branches from the brachial plexus. This bundle of vessels and nerves has its own fascial sheath, which houses and protects it.

The brachial and the antebrachial fasciae send out extensions to invest the various nerves and arteries as well as the deep and superficial veins in this region.

Antebrachial Fascia

The antebrachial fascia is continuous with the brachial fascia and terminates at the wrist where it is reinforced by the flexor and extensor retinaculae. To its superior part is attached an extension of the tendon of the biceps muscle. The anterior brachial and triceps muscles also send extensions from behind, which reinforce this tissue.

The fascia is thicker posteriorly than anteriorly. There are inferior insertion points at the level of the wrist (through the association of the retinaculae) and its posterior part is intimately associated with the posterior edge of the ulna. In addition, it sends out a second extension to the posterior edge of the radius which, together with elements of the skeleton, denote the anterior and posterior antebrachial regions.

From its deep face issue various muscular sheaths which invest the different muscles and provide a lubricating surface so they can easily slide over one another (Fig. 2-10). In the anterior region, the fascia divides to separate the superficial from the deep layer. The same arrangement is also observed in the posterior part.

The muscles invested by the antebrachial fascia can be divided into a series of different groups. The lateral group includes the long supinator muscle and both radial extensor muscles of the wrist; these three muscles all seem to be invested by the same fascial element, a fact of some significance, as becomes clear in clinical practice. The same arrangement applies to the medial part with the ulnar flexor and extensor muscles of the wrist, although in this case, the organization is less clear-cut.

Fig. 2-10 Forearm: Horizontal Cross-section at the One-third Distal Point

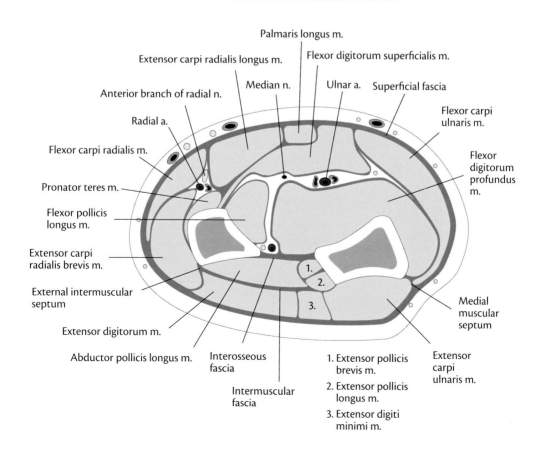

Fasciae of the Hand

The fasciae of the hand continue the antebrachial fascia distally from the retinaculae (Fig. 2-11). Distinction is made between two different fascial elements: the dorsal fascia of the hand and the palmar aponeurosis.

Fig. 2-11   Hand: Cross-section

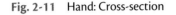

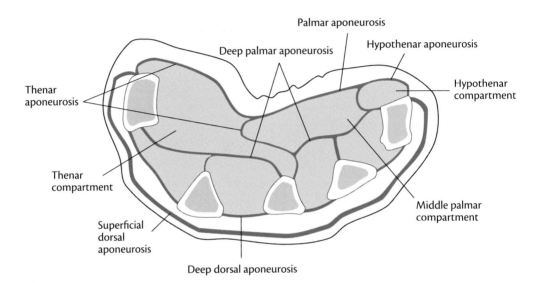

Dorsal fascia of the hand

Two different layers are usually considered: a superficial layer and a deep layer.

▶ SUPERFICIAL LAYER

The superficial layer is thin and covered by the extensor tendons. It is continuous with the extensor retinaculum and, at the bottom, with the extensor tendons. It is inserted at the phalanges. On the sides, it is inserted into the external edges of the first and fifth metacarpal bones.

▶ DEEP LAYER

The deep layer is very thin and covers the dorsal surface of the palmar interosseous muscles.

Palmar aponeurosis

Again, there are considered to be superficial and deep layers.

▶ SUPERFICIAL PALMAR APONEUROSIS

The superficial palmar aponeurosis consists of three sections: a middle part, or the true palmar aponeurosis, and two lateral elements which cover the thenar and hypothenar eminences.

▶ MIDDLE PALMAR APONEUROSIS

This is triangular in shape, with the base corresponding to the roots of the last four fingers. At the top, it is continuous with the antebrachial fascia and the flexor retinaculum and extends out as the tendon of the palmaris longus, which is the tensor of the aponeurosis. This is a strong fibrous band located just below the skin to which it is closely attached via short, fibrous extensions. Dupuytren described the presence of longer extensions, the cutaneous papillae, which start at the inferior third of the aponeurosis and extend as far as the interdigital fold. These papillae are maximally stretched during extension movements and it is the same structures which are responsible for the retraction of the palmar aponeurosis seen in Dupuyten's contracture.

The aponeurosis covers the flexor tendons, vessels, and nerves of the palm of the hand and is continuous on both sides with the aponeuroses of the thenar and hypothenar eminences (Fig. 2-12). It extends into the fingers to form sheaths for the flexor tendons, which are inserted into the phalanges. The middle palmar aponeurosis contains both longitudinal and transverse fibers.

Fig. 2-12 Middle and Deep Palmar Aponeuroses

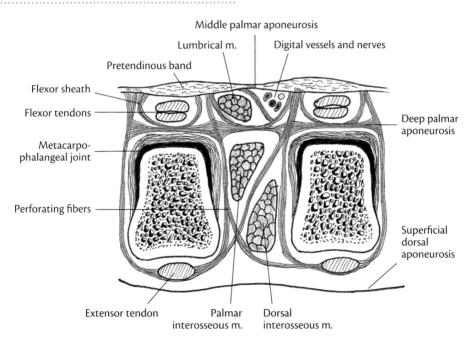

Longitudinal fibers. These continue out of the retinaculae and the tendon of the palmaris longus muscle. They descend, radiating out towards the four last fingers at the metacarpophalangeal articulations. They form eight slips, two for each of the four last fingers. These slips are attached to the lateral surfaces of the first phalanx of each finger and represent the most distal component of the superficial fascia of the upper limb.

Before the tendons, fibers come together to form pretendinous bands which join up with the thinner intratendinous membranes. The fibers in the pretendinous bands terminate in three different ways:

- some are attached to the deep layer of the skin
- others continue on to reach the deep aponeurosis. They form sagittally disposed septa which, together with the superficial and deep fasciae, define fascial tunnels. These tunnels variously invest the flexor tendons, the lumbrical muscles, and the vessels and nerves of the fingers.
- they send out penetrating fibers to the metacarpophalangeal articulation across the flexor retinaculum and around the joint to the extensor tendon behind which they join up with the similar fibers derived from the dorsum

Transverse fibers. The fasciae are covered by longitudinally oriented fibers at the inferior part of the aponeurosis which constitute the superficial transverse and interdigital ligaments.

▶ LATERAL PALMAR APONEUROSES

The lateral palmar aponeuroses are much thinner than the middle layer and they invest the muscles of the thenar and hypothenar eminences. Laterally, the external layer is inserted into the scaphoid and trapezium bones, and along the outer edge of the first metacarpal bone. Medially, it descends between the thenar muscles before attaching to the anterior edge of the third metacarpal. The medial layer is inserted into the pisiform bone and the medial edge of the fifth metacarpal. Laterally, it is inserted along the anterior edge of the fifth metacarpal. Thus, it forms a compartment for the hypothenar muscles.

▶ DEEP PALMAR APONEUROSIS

At the top, it is continuous with the fibrous elements of the wrist and terminates at the metacarpophalangeal articulations. In front of the heads of the second, third, fourth, and fifth metacarpals, the aponeurosis thickens to form the flexor retinaculum.

Table 2-2   Connections of the Upper Limb Fasciae

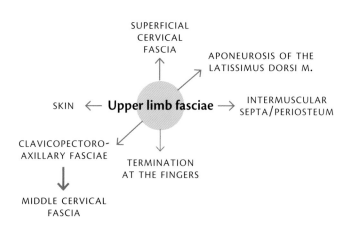

Summary of Upper Limb Fasciae

The fasciae of the upper limb are continuous with the superficial cervical fascia and articulate with the anterior and posterior thoracic fasciae.

They terminate in the fingers after having established strong connection at the elbow and the wrist.

Numerous veins, lymphatics, and nerves run over and pass through them.

These fasciae are composed of vertically and obliquely disposed fibers which interlace with one another and are woven together to create a particularly strong tissue.

A series of different membranes emanate from the deep surface of the fasciae:

- in a perpendicular direction: the intermuscular septa, which anchor it to the periosteum and then connect through to the osseous trabeculae;

- longitudinal membranes, which go on to invest the various muscles or form deep aponeurotic structures

Finally, the fascia of the upper limb splits repeatedly to invest and protect vessels and nerves, both superficially and deeply.

LOWER LIMB FASCIAE

The fascia of the lower limb is continuous with the lumbar and abdominal fasciae. The posterolateral part of this tissue originates in the iliac crest and at the sacrum where it extends the lumbosacral fascia and the sacrotuberous ligament. Its anterior portion originates from the pubis, the inferior pubic ramus, and the inguinal ligament. It terminates at the feet, having established relay points in the knee and the ankle. It is composed of interlacing vertical, horizontal, and oblique fibers.

The fascia wraps around the thigh and the leg from the top towards the bottom and from the outside towards the inside. The wrapping is more marked around the thigh. Whereas the fascia of the lower limb is thin posteromedially, it is thick anterolaterally and on the outside where it is referred to as the fascia lata . The fascia lata is the thickest and strongest fascia in the whole body. From its deep surface emanate many septa which will be dealt with in the order of the different segments of the lower limb.

Over its superficial surface (which is separated from the plane of the skin by the superficial fascia) run lymphatics, two major veins, and various sensory nerves (Fig. 2-13).

Fig. 2-13 Lower Limb Fasciae

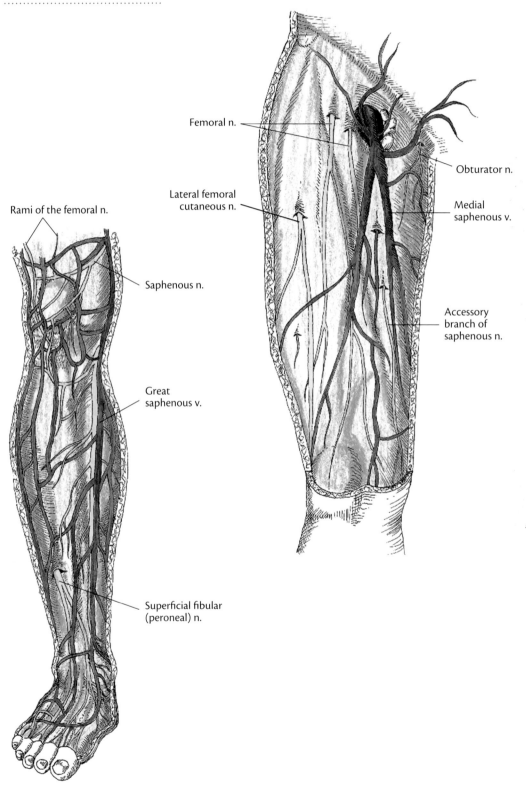

Femoral n.

Obturator n.

Lateral femoral
cutaneous n.

Medial
saphenous v.

Rami of the femoral n.

Saphenous n.

Accessory
branch of
saphenous n.

Great
saphenous v.

Superficial fibular
(peroneal) n.

Veins

The two largest veins are:

Small saphenous vein

The small saphenous vein originates at the external edge of the foot and then follows a course which is situated more or less towards the medial, posterior part of the leg. In most cases, it passes through the tibial fascia at the popliteal fossa to empty into the popliteal vein. It should be noted that this configuration can vary and this perforation of the tibial fascia can sometimes be found in the upper third of the calf, sometimes in the lower third, and sometimes even at the level of the Achilles tendon.

Great saphenous vein

The great saphenous vein originates at the medial edge of the foot, passes in front of the medial malleolus, and follows the medial side of the leg and thigh before passing through the cribriform fascia to empty into the femoral vein in the inguinal region. The cribriform fascia is attached to and sends an extension out over the tunica externa of the vein.

Cutaneous Nerves

From the top to bottom and from medial to lateral:

Anterior aspects

- the ilioinguinal nerve (in the inguinal region)
- the saphenous nerve, descending all the way down to the great toe, with an accessory branch in the most medial part which terminates at the medial aspect of the knee
- the internal obturator nerve on the medial surface as far as the knee
- the perforating cutaneous nerve in the medial part as far as the knee
- the crural branch of the genitofemoral nerve in the medial, superior part
- the lateral femoral cutaneous nerve in the lateral part
- the lateral sural cutaneous nerve of the calf and the superficial fibular nerve on the lateral part below the knee
- the superficial fibular nerve on the lateral leg and the superior, lateral foot

Posterior aspect

▶ AT THE BUTTOCKS

- the sacrococcygeal plexus medially
- the posterior cutaneous femoral nerve
- the first and second lumbar roots in the superior part
- a branch of the ilioinguinal nerve in the superior, medial part

The posterior and medial sides of the thigh are innervated by the posterior cutaneous femoral nerve as far as the popliteal fossa:

- the medial, posterior side is innervated by the saphenous and anterior cutaneous nerves
- the lateral, posterior side is innervated by the lateral cutaneous nerve

  ▶ IN THE CALF

- the sural nerve innervates the medial part
- the lateral cutaneous nerve of the calf (an accessory of the sural nerve) for the lateral, posterior part

Next, the various segments of the fascial system of the lower limb, its deep surface, and its numerous extensions will be discussed.

Gluteal Aponeurosis

The gluteal aponeurosis originates at the iliac crest, the sacrum, the coccyx, and the sacrotuberous ligament from which it extends inferiorly and anteriorly with the fascia lata. The anterior part of this fascia invests the gluteus medius muscle. When it reaches the anterior edge of the gluteus maximus muscle, it divides to form superficial, middle, and deep layers.

The superficial and middle layers invest the superficial and deep surfaces of the gluteus maximus muscle. The deep layer is highly cellular. It invests successively (superior to inferior):

- the posterior part of the gluteus medius muscle
- the piriformis muscle
- the gemellus muscles
- the quadratus femoris muscle of the thigh

It is interrupted:

- above the piriformis muscle in order to allow the passage of vessels and nerves supplying the superior glutei muscles
- below the piriformis muscle in order to allow the passage of the sciatic vessels and the sciatic nerve

Finally, two cellular membranes invest the deep surface of the gluteus medius muscle and the external surface of the gluteus minimus muscle. These two membranes are continuous with the deep layer of the gluteal aponeurosis across the entire length of the fascial plane which separates the gluteus medius from the piriformis muscle (Fig. 2-14).

For this reason, the gluteal aponeurosis divides to form several different membranes to cover all of the various muscles. These membranes allow the different muscles to slide over one another. They also define cleavage planes, which we can utilize for deep palpation. Notably, we can access the piriformis and gemellus muscles via the plane between the gluteus medius and the gluteus maximus muscles. These will be discussed in Chapters 7 and 8 below.

Fig. 2-14 Horizontal Cross-section through the Adductor Canal in the Thigh

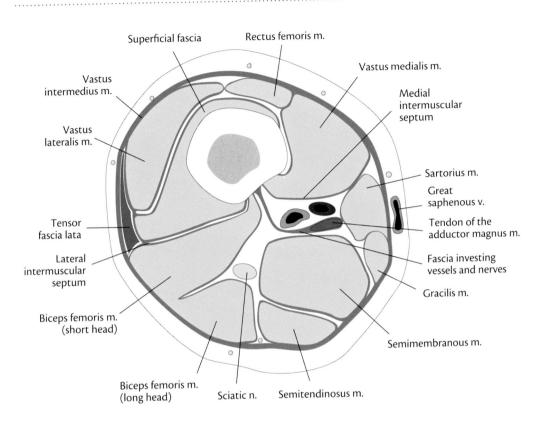

Fasciae of the Thigh

Superiorly, the fascia lata is attached to the pubis at the inguinal ligament and to the ischiopubic ramus. Posterolaterally, it is continuous with the gluteal aponeurosis. This fascia extends down into the tibial aponeurosis with several points of attachment to the patella, the intercondylar eminence, and the head of the fibula.

The organization of the medial, superior part of the fascia of the thigh around the femoral triangle is somewhat specialized and this fascial element is usually distinguished as the cribriform fascia. Here, the tissue is thin, loose, and pierced to allow for the passage of the great number of lymphatic vessels making their way from the superficial to deeper layers. The most remarkable of all these openings is that which exists for the great saphenous vein: around the periphery of this opening the fascia thickens to form a ring, called the saphenous opening (fossa ovalis), to which the sheath of the vein is attached.

This cribriform fascia is itself a aponeurotic fold which allows adduction and internal rotation of the thigh without exerting excessive tension on the fascia, which might result in damage to the vessels and nerves. Its superficial surface splits to invest the sartorius muscle. Extensions project from its deep surface which invest each of the various muscles of the thigh. The fascia lata is linked to the femur through two septa, the medial and lateral intermuscular septa (Fig. 2-14).

Medial intermuscular septum

This septum extends down from an oblique line drawn from the greater and the lesser trochanter to the medial condyle of the knee. It is attached to the medial edge of the linea aspera and its lower part contributes to the adductor hiatus of the adductor magnus muscle, through which passes the femoral artery. Its thick, prominent medial edge is easy to palpate (it feels like a cord). Distally, it seems to be continuous with the medial collateral ligament of the knee. Its anterior surface is inserted into the vastus medialis muscle and its posterior surface is in contact with the adductor muscles. It is strongly attached to the aponeuroses of these muscles.

On the inside of the anterior thigh this fascia divides to form two compartments:

- a lateral, anterior compartment which contains the quadriceps muscles
- a medial, posterior compartment which contains the adductor muscles, the gracilis muscle and the femoral vessels

A thin septum separates the medial, posterior compartment from the posterior one.

Lateral intermuscular septum

This septum extends down from the greater trochanter to the lateral condyle of the femur. Above the lateral condyle, and after insertion into the lateral lip of the linea aspera femoris, it takes the form of a prominent cord. Anteriorly it serves as an insertion point for the vastus lateralis muscle and posteriorly for the short portion of the biceps femoris muscle. It separates the anterior and posterior compartments.

Sheath of the femoral vessels

The fascia lata splits to form a sheath which invests and protects the femoral vessels. This sheath extends from the inguinal ligament to the adductor foramen; the superior part of this canal is called the femoral canal, and the inferior part is called the adductor (or Hunter's) canal. This canal is in the shape of a triangular prism which has been twisted along its axis so that the surface which is initially anterior becomes the medial surface at the bottom.

Here again, this twisted configuration of the fascia protects the vessels and nerves of the femoral canal (including the femoral artery and vein, and the saphenous nerve and its accessory) from compression and stretching when the thigh is moved, especially during external rotation and abduction. An extra element contributes to the protection of this canal by investing its inferior part, namely, the sartorius muscle, which has a similar obliquely spiral trajectory as it passes inferomedially.

Fascia of the Lower Leg

The fascia of the lower leg is directly continuous with the posterior part of the fascia lata femoris after insertion into the patella, the tibial condyles, and the anterior part of the head of the fibula. Here it is also attached to the tendons of the biceps femoris on the outside and the sartorius and the semitendinosus muscle on the inside. A series of different membranes issue from its deep side and then proceed to invest muscles and form the medial and lateral intermuscular septa (Fig. 2-15).

Fig. 2-15   Cross-section through the Middle Third of the Leg

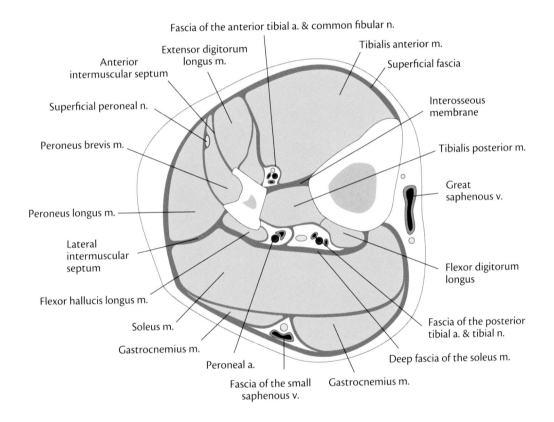

Posterior intermuscular septum

The posterior intermuscular septum extends from the internal surface of the aponeurosis at the lateral edge of the fibula. This septum separates the lateral, anterior region from the posterior region.

Anterior intermuscular septum

The anterior intermuscular septum extends from the deep surface of the aponeurosis at the anterior edge of the fibula and divides the lateral, anterior leg into an anterior compartment and a lateral compartment that contains the peroneal muscles.

The anterior compartment contains the extensor hallucis longus and the tibialis anterior muscles, both of which are inserted in the tibial aponeurosis. This compartment also contains the common extensor muscles of the toes.

At the head of the tibia there is an osteofibromuscular structure, formed by the tendinous arch of the soleus muscle with the posterior tibia, which invests the sciatic nerve and has the ability to compress it. On the lateral, anterior side of the leg, the tibial aponeurosis directly invests the tibia and is strongly attached to its periosteum.

At the level of the popliteal fossa, the posterior part of the tibial aponeurosis splits to invest the deep muscles and the various vessels and nerves, separating them from the soleus and gastrocnemius muscles, known collectively as the triceps surae. This allows them to slide easily over the deeper structures.

Fascial Elements of the Foot

On the dorsum, the fascial system of the foot is continuous with the tibial aponeurosis via the retinaculum, and on the plantar surface, it terminates at the toes (Fig. 2-16). Distinction is usually made between the dorsal and the plantar aponeuroses.

Fig. 2-16 Vertical Cross-section through the Foot

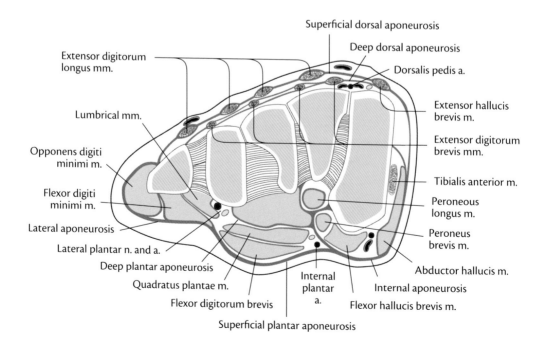

Superficial dorsal aponeurosis

Deep dorsal aponeurosis

Extensor digitorum longus mm.

Dorsalis pedis a.

Lumbrical mm.

Extensor hallucis brevis m.

Opponens digiti minimi m.

Extensor digitorum brevis mm.

Flexor digiti minimi m.

Tibialis anterior m.

Lateral aponeurosis

Peroneous longus m.

Lateral plantar n. and a.

Peroneus brevis m.

Deep plantar aponeurosis

Abductor hallucis m.

Quadratus plantae m.

Internal plantar a.

Internal aponeurosis

Flexor digitorum brevis

Flexor hallucis brevis m.

Superficial plantar aponeurosis

Dorsal aponeuroses

These are three in number:

▶ SUPERFICIAL APONEUROSIS

This aponeurosis invests the extensor tendons. On the sides it is attached to the medial and lateral edges of the foot where it is continuous with the plantar aponeurosis.

▶ APONEUROSIS OF THE SHORT EXTENSOR MUSCLES OF THE TOES

This corresponds to a division of the superficial aponeurosis. It invests the short extensor muscles of the toes, the vessels of the foot, and the anterior tibial nerve. Laterally it is inserted into the lateral edge of the foot, and medially it is continuous with the superficial aponeurosis.

▶ DEEP APONEUROSIS

This emanates from the extensor retinaculum and invests the dorsal surface of the metatarsals and the interosseous muscles.

Plantar aponeuroses

There are two plantar aponeuroses, one superficial and the other deep.

▶ SUPERFICIAL PLANTAR APONEUROSIS

This aponeurosis is separated from the skin by a thick layer of adipose tissue and, like the superficial palmar aponeurosis, can be divided into three different compartments:

- a central compartment
- a medial compartment
- a lateral compartment

Central compartment. This is an extremely strong membrane which is thick all over, but especially in its posterior aspect. It helps maintain the longitudinal arches of the foot. This aponeurosis corresponds to a triangle which radiates out anteriorly from its points of attachment at the metatarsalphalangeal articulations to the calcaneal tuberosity posteriorly. It contains very strong, longitudinally disposed fibers which form pretendinous bands anteriorly. These are superimposed with transversely oriented fibers, especially in the anterior part; at the metacarpophalangeal articulations, these latter fibers form superficial transverse ligaments which support the anterior plantar arch. On the sides it is continuous with the lateral and medial aponeuroses.

Medial compartment. This tissue is much thinner than the central plantar aponeurosis and extends from the medial tubercle of the calcaneum to the root of the great toe. On the outside it is continuous with the middle aponeurosis, and on the inside with the superficial plantar aponeurosis.

Lateral compartment. Posteriorly this aponeurosis is attached to the lateral tubercle of the calcaneus; anteriorly it attaches to the fifth metacarpal. On the inside it is continuous with the middle aponeurosis, and on the outside with the superficial aponeurosis.

At the point where the middle aponeurosis continues through into the lateral and medial aponeuroses, it sends out sagittal extensions which attach:

- medially to the navicular bone, first cuneiform bone, and the inferior surface of the first metacarpal
- laterally to the sheath of the long peroneal muscle and the fifth metacarpal

These septa form three separate compartments on the plantar side of the foot: a medial, a middle, and a lateral compartment. None of these compartments is sealed and they are crossed by numerous vessels and nerves.

► DEEP APONEUROSIS

The deep aponeurosis invests the interosseous muscles. Posteriorly, it terminates in the form of fibrous components of the tarsus, and anteriorly, it is continuous with the deep transverse metatarsal ligament.

It should be remembered that, in the lower limb as in the upper limb, the tibial fascia repeatedly divides to invest the various superficial and deep components of the vascular and nervous systems. Most notably, this includes the sciatic nerve which, together with its many branches, is invested with a fascial sheath throughout its entire length down through the common, superficial, and deep fibular nerves. As will be seen later, this sheath is often involved in pathology affecting this nerve.

Table 2-3   Connections of the Lower Limb Fasciae

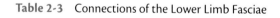

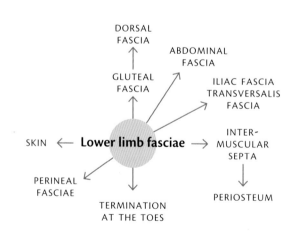

Summary of Lower Limb Fasciae

This system is continuous with the fascia of the trunk through the gluteal aponeurosis.

It is attached at the knee and the ankles, and terminates in the foot.

It supports a complex network of veins, lymphatics, and nerves which regularly perforate its surface.

It is composed of vertical, oblique, and horizontal fibers which are woven together and interlace to generate an extremely strong tissue.

A series of different membranes emanate from its deep surface:
- in a perpendicular direction, the intermuscular septa, which anchor the fascia to the periosteum and from there continue through the osseous trabeculae
- longitudinal membranes, which go on to invest the various muscles or form deep aponeurotic structures

Finally, the fascia of the upper limb splits repeatedly to invest and protect vessels and nerves, both superficially and deeply.

It also articulates with:
- the thoracic fascia
- the superficial and deep perineal fasciae via the aponeuroses of the piriformis and internal obturator muscles
- the iliac fascia via the aponeurosis of the psoas muscle
- and finally, the deep abdominal fascia and the transversalis fascia at the inguinal ligament

Internal Fasciae

The internal fasciae will be dealt with in the following order:
- the fasciae of the neck (the cervical and prevertebral fasciae)
- the fasciae of the thorax
- the fasciae of the abdomen
- the fasciae of the pelvis

MIDDLE CERVICAL FASCIA

The middle cervical fascia extends from the hyoid bone to the posterior face of the clavicle and the sternum. Its sides invest the omohyoid muscles and it is continuous with the superficial and deep fasciae at the anterior edge of the trapezius muscle (Fig. 2-17).

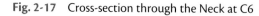

Fig. 2-17   Cross-section through the Neck at C6

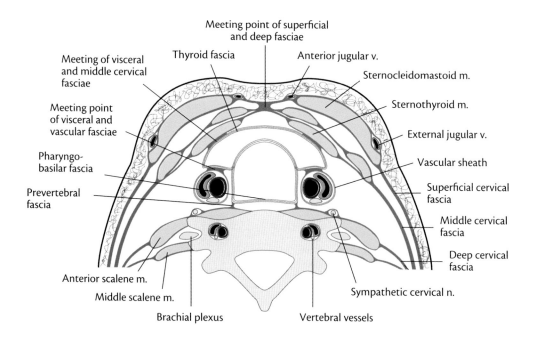

Meeting point of superficial and deep fasciae

Thyroid fascia

Anterior jugular v.

Meeting of visceral and middle cervical fasciae

Sternocleidomastoid m.

Sternothyroid m.

Meeting point of visceral and vascular fasciae

External jugular v.

Pharyngo-basilar fascia

Vascular sheath

Prevertebral fascia

Superficial cervical fascia

Middle cervical fascia

Deep cervical fascia

Anterior scalene m.

Middle scalene m.

Sympathetic cervical n.

Brachial plexus

Vertebral vessels

In the front, the middle cervical fascia is joined to the superficial fascia as far as the lower end of the larynx. Lower down, the two fasciae separate to define the substernal space through which passes the anterior jugular vein.

At the level of the anterior neck muscles, the middle cervical fascia splits into a superficial sheet for the sternocleidomastoid and omohyoid muscles, and a deep sheet for the thyrohyoid and sternothyroid muscles.

Expansions project from its deep face which connect with the peripharyngeal membrane and the vascular bundle of the neck which surrounds the common carotid artery, the internal jugular vein, and the vagus nerve, each component being invested with its own sheath. It also sends out an extension to the thyroid gland and contributes to the fascia of that organ.

In the inferior, lateral part, after attachment to the clavicle, are extremely strong extensions to the brachiocephalic venous trunk and the subclavian vein, which keep these veins open and in place. They also contribute to the subclavian fascia.

The middle cervical fascia extends down into the anterior thorax in the form of the endothoracic fascia.

PREVERTEBRAL FASCIA

The front of this fascia invests the prevertebral muscles of the neck, hence its alternate name, nuchal fascia. It is attached:

- superiorly to the basilar apophysis of the occipital bone
- laterally to the transverse processes of the cervical vertebrae where it is continuous with the apneurosis of the scalenes. Through this it joins with both the deep face of the superficial fascia in front of the anterior edge of the trapezius muscle, and the middle cervical fascia. In this way, it separates the visceral sheath in front from the muscular sheath of the neck behind.

Anteriorly on the median line, it is connected to the pharynx and the esophagus via a very loose sheet of cellular tissue. Laterally it extends to the carotid arteries, the internal jugular vein, and the vagus nerve, as well as to the anterior branches of the spinal nerves which are invested by the prevertebral fasciae.

Posteriorly, extensions of this fascia invest the prevertebral muscles: the longus colli muscle of the neck and the rectus capitis anterior muscles (both minor and major). It should be noted that these muscles are the only suboccipital muscles to be located in front of the vertebral column and are therefore within the cavity. It also supports the sympathetic nerves and communicating branches which are held in a continuation of the prevertebral fascia or in a special sheath. After insertion in the first thoracic vertebra, it continues down in the form of the posterior endothoracic fascia (Fig. 2-18).

ENDOTHORACIC FASCIA

The endothoracic fascia lines the inner surface of the thoracic cage, lying interior to the ribs and the internal intercostal muscles to which it is attached via fibrous connections (Fig. 2-19). Behind, as Rouviere has shown, opposite the lateral face of the vertebral column, the endothoracic fascia is denser and is attached to the vertebrae via fine ligaments.

Higher up, the endothoracic fascia covers the pleural dome and is attached to the periosteum of the first rib, especially strongly to its posterior portion. In addition, in front, it is also attached to the sheath of the subclavian artery (establishing a link with the cervical fascia). Here it thickens significantly to form a fibrous transverse septum within which separate ligaments which suspend the pleura are distinguished:

- the costopleural ligament
- the transverse cupular ligament
- the pleurovertebral ligament

Its lower part covers the diaphragm to which it is very tightly attached and by means of which it extends down into the abdominal wall through the fascia transversalis. Its inner face is strongly attached to the parietal pleura, which is thereby attached to the thoracic wall. It is thick and relatively soft around the mediastinum, although it changes into a fibrous layer where it is joined to the pericardium immediately underneath the pleura.

The pleura attaches to the thoracic wall by means of the endothoracic fascia:

anteriorly it does so at the sternum, and posteriorly between the posterior angle of the ribs and the vertebral column, and also to the vertebral column itself.

Summary of the Fascia of the Neck

1. A superficial fascia which extends downward from the cranial fasciae and terminates around the thoracic outlet, continuous with the fasciae of the:
   – thorax
   – upper limbs.

   • It invests the superficial muscles, nerves, and veins of the anterior and posterior neck.

   • It is continuous with the middle cervical and prevertebral fasciae at the lateral edge of the trapezius muscle in the anterior neck.

2. A middle fascia present in the anterolateral part of the neck which originates at the hyoid bone, passes down through the sternum, and continues into the endothoracic fascia.

   • It invests the deep anterior, lateral muscles.

   • It invests the neurovascular bundle (the carotid vessels, the jugular vein, and the vagus nerve) which pass through the neck.

   • It goes on to be part of the thyrolaryngeal fascia.

   • It connects with the superficial and deep fasciae, and with the pharyngobasilar fascia.

3. A deep fascia.

   • This originates in the basilar apophysis of the occiput.

   • It extends downward via the endothoracic fascia after insertion into T_1.

   • Posteriorly, it is attached to the transverse processes of the cervical vertebrae.

   • It forms the scalene fascia and through this joins the middle and superficial fasciae, and invests the prevertebral muscles.

   • It supports the cervical plexus and, in the form of an extension, the cervical ganglia.

   • Finally, it is connected to the pharyngobasilar fascia by anteroposterior membranes.

Fig. 2-18   Sagittal Section Showing the Fasciae of the Neck

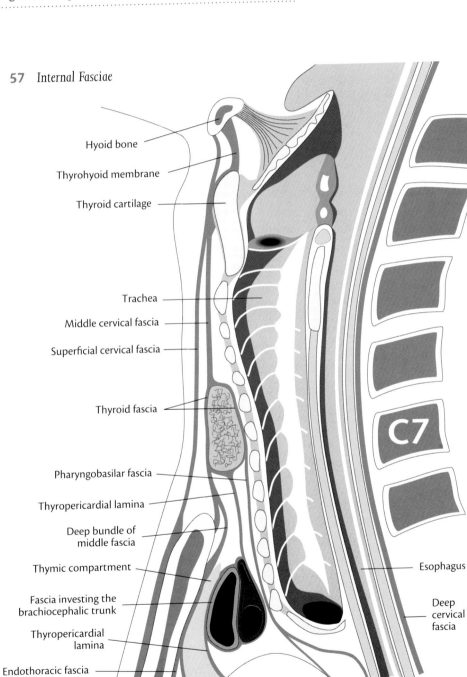

57   *Internal Fasciae*

Hyoid bone

Thyrohyoid membrane

Thyroid cartilage

Trachea

Middle cervical fascia

Superficial cervical fascia

Thyroid fascia

Pharyngobasilar fascia

Thyropericardial lamina

Deep bundle of middle fascia

Thymic compartment

Fascia investing the brachiocephalic trunk

Thyropericardial lamina

Endothoracic fascia

Superior sterno-pericardial lig.

C7

Esophagus

Deep cervical fascia

2-19   Vertical Section through the Thoracic Wall

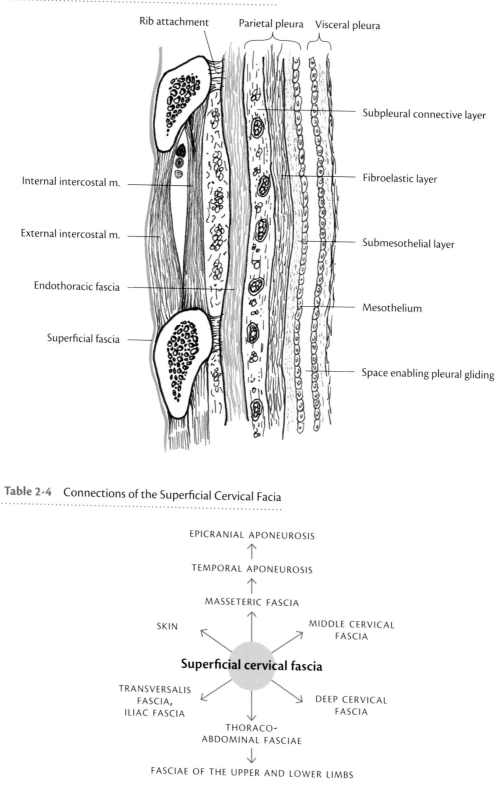

Rib attachment   Parietal pleura   Visceral pleura

Subpleural connective layer

Internal intercostal m.

Fibroelastic layer

External intercostal m.

Submesothelial layer

Endothoracic fascia

Mesothelium

Superficial fascia

Space enabling pleural gliding

Table 2-4   Connections of the Superficial Cervical Facia

EPICRANIAL APONEUROSIS

TEMPORAL APONEUROSIS

MASSETERIC FASCIA

SKIN   MIDDLE CERVICAL
                                        FASCIA

Superficial cervical fascia

TRANSVERSALIS
FASCIA,   DEEP CERVICAL
ILIAC FASCIA   FASCIA

THORACO-
ABDOMINAL FASCIAE

FASCIAE OF THE UPPER AND LOWER LIMBS

Table 2-5 Connections of the Middle Cervical Fascia

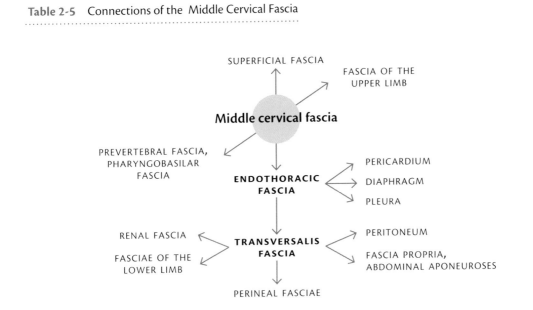

Table 2-6 Connections of the Deep Cervical Fascia

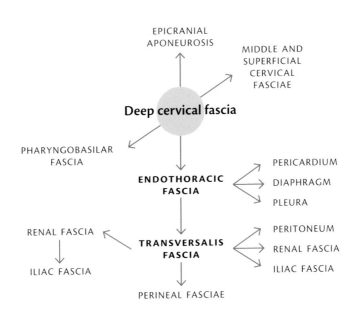

TRANSVERSALIS FASCIA

The transversalis fascia lines the inner surface of the abdomen. It adheres tightly to the parietal peritoneum via the fascia propria and it is difficult to distinguish the two. Its lower part splits to form a sac surrounding the kidney. This sac is formed from a retrorenal fascia, the middle part of which is attached behind to the major vessels and the vertebrae, and from a prerenal fascia. These two fasciae join on the sides in front to form the sac which contains the kidneys. The top of this fascia is attached to the diaphragm, and the bottom to the iliac fascia.

Its lower part is in contact with the organs of the lesser pelvis and is continuous with the parietal peritoneum. It extends a diverticulum into the inguinal canal, which forms the fibrous sheath of the cord. The transversalis fascia is also continuous with the sheath of the external iliac arteries. In its anterior and middle parts, it is strengthened by the inguinal falx (Henle's ligament) and the interfoveolar (Hesselbach's) ligament.

Posteriorly it originates at the lateral edge of the lumbar region where it is connected to the iliac fascia: its ventral portion is intimately associated with the

Summary of the Endothoracic and Transversalis Fasciae

These correspond to continuations of the fasciae of the neck. The cervical and prevertebral fasciae continue to form the endothoracic fascia, which itself continues to form the transversalis fascia after a detour to create the diaphragm.

The endothoracic fascia connects:

- on the outside, with the inner surface of the thoracic cavity

- on the inside, with the pleura and the pericardium

- inferiorly, with the diaphragm and then the transversalis fascia

The transversalis fascia joins:

- superiorly, with the diaphragm and the endothoracic fascia

- on the outside, with the deep abdominal fasciae and the renal fascia

- interiorly, with the peritoneum

- inferiorly, with the fasciae of the lesser pelvis of, on the one hand, the lower limb and, on the other hand, its extensions toward the inguinal ligament (forming a channel of communication to the outside) linea alba. It is formed of transverse fibers plus, especially in its anterior portion, vertical and obliquely inclined fibers. It varies in thickness, being thickest in the subumbilical part.

The anterolateral part of the fascia transversalis is in contact with the abdominal fasciae from which its posterior part is separated by the renal fascia. This, as discussed in the previous section, rests on the iliac fascia, which itself results from the splitting of the posterior abdominal fasciae.

The iliac fascia is attached medially to the vertebral bodies, and to the insertion of the psoas muscle on the inominate bone. Laterally it is attached to the quadratus lumborum.

Higher up, the iliac fascia is thickened at what is known as the medial arcuate ligament, a tendinous arch in the fascia that covers the superior part of the psoas muscle. On the inside, this is attached to the body of the second lumbar vertebra and then passes around the psoas in front to terminate at the base of the transverse process of the first lumbar vertebra.

The iliac fascia is attached to the inguinal ligament in front, while its medial part is thickened to form a strong, fibrous lamella, the ileopectineal ligament, which defines the outer edge of the femoral ring. Below the arch, the iliac fascia extends to the trochanteric insertion of the iliopsoas and contributes to the fascia lata.

FASCIAE OF THE PERINEUM AND PELVIS

The perineal fasciae serve to close the lower part of the abdominal cavity. These very strong fasciae are inserted around the perimeter of the pelvis and contain openings in the anteroposterior direction. In the anterior part, there are necessarily differences between males and females.

They support and reinforce the three muscular planes of the lesser pelvis and are therefore three in number:

- the superficial fascia of the perineum
- the middle fascia of the perineum
- the deep fascia of the perineum, or urogenital diaphragm

Superficial Perineal Fascia

This subcutaneous fascia extends only as far as the anterior perineum. Its attachments are:

- on the sides, to the anterior lip of the ischiopubic rami
- superiorly, as it extends anteriorly, it is continuous with the superficial fascia of the penis in men. In women, it disappears on the inside in the connective tissue of the labia minora anteriorly, and is continuous with the fascia of the clitoris
- Its base extends from one ischium to the other and defines the border between the anterior and posterior perineum. Here, it curves posteriorly upwards and, having skirted the posterior edge of the superficial

transverse muscle, it joins with the lower sheet of the middle fascia. It sends extensions out to the central tendon of the perineum (Figs. 2-20 & 2-21).

- Extensions emanating from its deep surface line the deep perineal fascia as well as the ischiocavernosus and bulbospongiosus muscles. These extensions are fused with the deep sheet of the middle fascia.

Fig. 2-20   Fasciae of the Pelvis (Female)

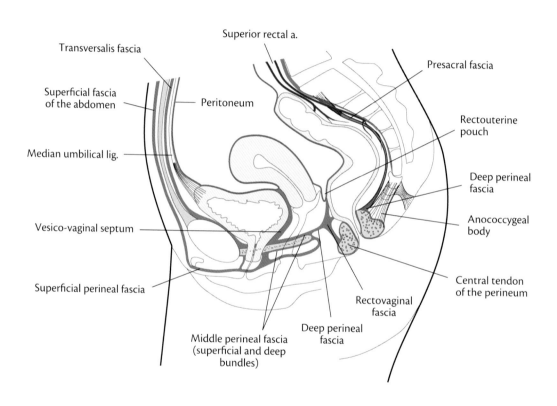

Middle Perineal Fascia

This structure is also known as the urogenital diaphragm or Cruveilhier's fascia. Triangular in shape, it only occupies the anterior, or urogenital triangle, of the perineum. Many different, sometimes contradictory descriptions have been published by, among others, Grégoire and Rouviere. This is evidence of the complexity of this fascial element. In our opinion, the clearest and most useful understanding of the anatomy here is that described by Testut and Rouvière.

This fascia consists of two layers, one below the muscles of the middle plane and the other above; the deep transverse perineal muscles are situated behind the fascia, and the urethra is in front.

Fig. 2-21   Frontal View of the Male Pelvis Sectioned through the Ischiopubic Rami

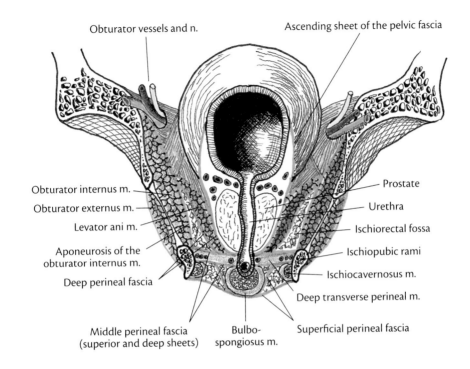

Obturator vessels and n.

Ascending sheet of the pelvic fascia

Obturator internus m.

Obturator externus m.

Levator ani m.

Aponeurosis of the obturator internus m.

Deep perineal fascia

Prostate

Urethra

Ischiorectal fossa

Ischiopubic rami

Ischiocavernosus m.

Deep transverse perineal m.

Middle perineal fascia (superior and deep sheets)

Bulbo-spongiosus m.

Superficial perineal fascia

Inferior layer

This thick, strong fascial layer, also known as the puboprostatic, perineal, or Carcassonne's ligament, inserts laterally into the medial surface of the ischium and into the internal lip of the lower edge of the ischiopubic ramus immediately below the attachments of the corpus cavernosum and the ischiocavernosus muscles. Its anterior (but not its posterior) part is attached to the ischiocavernous muscles. It extends transversally and, along the median line, is tightly associated with the dense fibrous tissue around the corpus spongiosum and the urethra.

Its posterior edge joins the superficial fascia of the perineum inferiorly, and the deep layer of the middle fascia superiorly. Posteriorly, it sends out extensions to the central tendon of the perineum. Anteriorly, it is continuous with the superior layer. The lower layer of the middle perineal fascia creates a secure attachment between the bulb and the corpus spongiosum of the penis, which it securely anchors to the ischiopubic rami.

Its nature is not the same throughout. Posteriorly, where it invests the deep transverse perineal muscle, it is thin, while it is thicker and stronger close to the membranous urethra. At this point the fascia resembles a ligament. Further anterior, it is thicker and continues to form the inferior pubic (arcuate) ligament, which closes the superior, anterior part of the perineum.

Superior layer

This layer covers the superior surface of the deep transverse perineal muscle and of the striated sphincter of the urethra. For this reason it is also known as the deep layer. Posteriorly, it joins the superficial layer of the fascia and sends extensions out towards the central tendon of the perineum (Fig. 2-22).

Its extreme anterior part unites with the inferior layer to form the inguinal aponeurotic fold, also known as the conjoined tendon, finally terminating at the arcuate ligament of pubis.

On the sides, the superior layer of the middle perineal fascia is attached to the ischiopubic ramus above the insertion point of the deep transverse muscle. It sends out an extension to the aponeurosis of the internal obturator. This extension splits to form a fibrous conduit, known as the pudendal canal or Alcock's canal, through which pass the pudendal vessels and nerves.

Fig. 2-22 Superficial and Middle Perineal Fascia

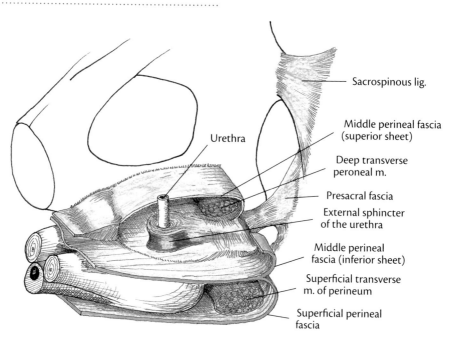

Sacrospinous lig.

Middle perineal fascia (superior sheet)

Urethra

Deep transverse peroneal m.

Presacral fascia

External sphincter of the urethra

Middle perineal fascia (inferior sheet)

Superficial transverse m. of perineum

Superficial perineal fascia

The posterior part of the middle fascia of the perineum has a lamella which ascends between the prostate and the membranous urethra in front and the rectum behind. At the top, it hangs from the rectouterine (females) or the rectovesical (males) pouch, which is also known as Douglas' pouch. It forms the rectovesical septum, also known as Denonvilliers aponeurosis.

This fascia splits into two membranes:

- a posterior membrane which forms the rectovesical septum
- an anterior membrane which invests the seminal vesicles, the vas deferensl, and the posterior portion of the prostate. Therefore, it forms

the prostatic cavity with the anterior part derived from the middle fascia of the perineum

In females, the rectovesical septum is replaced by a thin membranous lamella which forms the rectovaginal septum. In males, the two layers of the middle fascia of the perineum enclose the bulbourethral (Cowper's) glands. This contains two openings:

- the opening of the dorsal vein of the penis, between the arcuate ligament of pubis and the transverse inguinal falx
- further posterior is the opening of the membranous portion of the urethra, with its external sphincter situated even further posterior

Deep Fascia of the Perineum

This is a far more extensive fascia than the two that were previously discussed. It extends into both the anterior and posterior perineum, and even beyond the confines of the perineal region, to climb back up the lateral walls of the pelvis and reach parts of the superior aperture of the minor pelvis (Fig. 2-23).

Fig. 2-23 Frontal View of the Male Pelvis Sectioned through the Anus

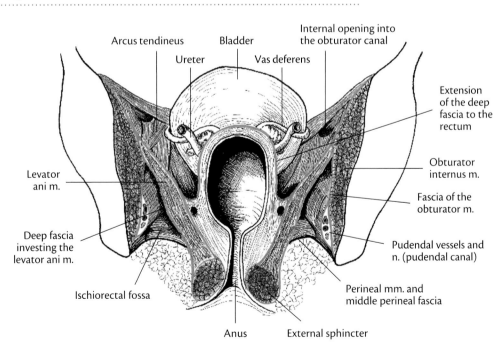

The superior part of the pelvic cavity contains eight muscles:

- the levator ani muscles in the central part
- the ischiococcygeal muscles behind
- the obturator muscles on the side
- the piriformis muscles in the posterolateral part

These eight muscles are each invested by a specific fascia. All these fasciae come together to form the deep perineal fascia which, together with the action of the above-mentioned muscles, close all the perineal openings apart from those in the median plane. Thus, the extensive perineal fascial system has the overall shape of a funnel. In order to facilitate description, it can be divided into two symmetrical halves, both of which can be considered independently in terms of:

- a lateral edge
- a medial edge
- a superior surface
- an inferior surface

Lateral edge

The lateral edge inserts:

- anteriorly, on the posterior surface of the body of the pubis and the horizontal ramus (connecting with the anterior abdominal fascia)
- on the fibrous arch which defines the bottom of the medial opening of the obturator canal and to which it contributes
- behind this same canal, it climbs back up as far as the pelvic inlet and inserts at the arcuate line where it fuses with the iliac fascia (connecting with the lateral abdominal and the pelvic fascial systems)
- it then descends toward the greater sciatic notch along the superior edge of the piriformis muscle
- finally, it arrives in contact with the presacral aponeruosis and attaches inside the anterior aspects of the sacral foramina (connecting with the abdominal fascia)

Medial edge

The two halves of the pelvic fascia only contact one another at two points on the median line:

- perineal raphe
- anococcygeal raphe

Anterior to the perineal raphe, they are separated by a triangular space formed by the middle fascia of the perineum. Between the two raphes, two halves of the pelvic fascia are separated by the rectal opening and join up again at the fibrous sheath of the pelvic rectum. At the level of the prostate, it unites with the lateral aponeurosis of the prostate, and through this link, with the middle fascia.

Inferior surface

The inferior surface rests directly on the underlying muscles and is joined to them by a thin layer of cellular tissue.

Superior surface

The superior surface is separated from the peritoneum by a space which contains the urethra, the vas deferens, and the vessels and nerves which supply the pelvic viscera. The deep perineal fascia is not of uniform thickness but contains three thickened ligamentous areas which radiate out from the ischial ridge to form a three-pointed star:

- the tendinous arch of the levator ani, which extends to the ischium
- a band of reinforcement which runs along the anterior edge of the greater sciatic notch of ischium
- a band of reinforcement which descends down along the junction of the coccygeal muscle on one side, and the piriformis along with the sacral plexus on the other

It should be noted that the aponeurosis of the obturator internus muscle—the superior part of which is associated with the middle and superior fasciae of the perineum—continues down through the sacrotuberous ligament and extends onto the anterior surface of the gluteus maximus muscle, which extends below this ligament (joining with the superficial fascia).

The deep perineal fascia sends out extensions to the central tendinous point of the perineum. In the anteroposterior direction, it is perforated by the rectum (surrounded by its sphincter), the urethra (at its exit point from the prostate), and in women, the vagina. The deep perineal fascia is inserted all around the periphery of the vagina and is one of the main structures supporting it.

The deep perineal fascia is attached to the colon via extensions (continuous with the visceral fascia), and its posterolateral part (the fascia investing the piriformis muscles) supports the lumbosacral plexus.

Other fascial elements are present in the pelvis and compartmentalize it by dividing the front from the back. The following will be considered in detail:

- the presacral aponeurosis
- the rectovesical or rectovaginal septa (previously mentioned)
- the vesicovaginal septum and the parametrium in females
- the umbilical ligaments
- the sacrogenital folds along with the membranes covering the internal iliac artery and hypogastric plexus

The first four structures are vascular membranes oriented in the frontal plane. The last septum has a sagittal orientation.

Related Perineal Fascial Structures

Presacral aponeurosis

This aponeurosis descends from the abdomen with the middle rectal artery (it is continuous with the abdominal fasciae), lining the interior surface of the sacrum. It joins the posterior surface of the rectum via its fibrous sheath, which is called the retrorectal fascia. The retrorectal fascia extends from the termination of the sigmoid mesocolon down as far as the floor of the pelvis.

The posterior part of the deep perineal fascia terminates at this structure, which supports the lamella of the sacrogenital folds. It also supports the sacral plexus and the coccygeal body.

Rectovesical and rectovaginal septa

See previous discussion.

Vesicovaginal aponeurosis

The bladder is separated from the vagina by a cellular septum, the vesicovaginal fascia. The juxtavesical terminal segment of the ureter transversely crosses the thickness of this fascia. The rectovaginal and vesicovaginal septa extend to the broad ligament of the uterus, which is a thickened part of the peritoneum investing the uterus, the fallopian tubes, the ovaries, and the round ligaments of the uterus (Fig. 2-24). This ligament has a very complicated shape and only a brief description will be given.

Fig. 2-24   Arrangement of the Pelvic Fasciae

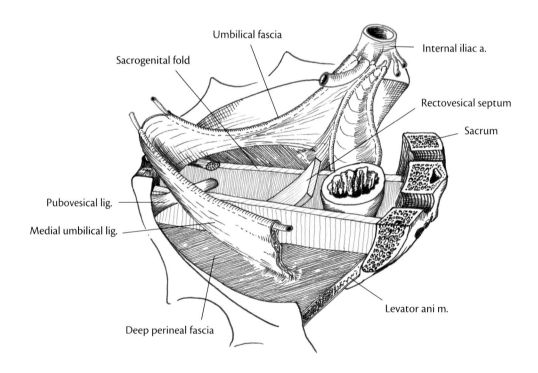

The broad ligament of the uterus is formed by two peritoneal sheets which line, respectively, the anterior and posterior surfaces of the organ. Starting from the lateral edge of the uterus, these two juxtaposed sheets (which are continuous with one another) pass outwards to reach the lateral wall of the pelvis, where they fold back to form the pelvic parietal peritoneum. In a similar fashion, at the bottom, the two sheets begin to spread away from one another as they move back across the floor of the pelvis. Where they fold back, one turns forward and the other turns back to form the pelvic peritoneum of the base of the pelvis (Fig. 2-25).

Fig. 2-25   Superior View of Female Pelvis

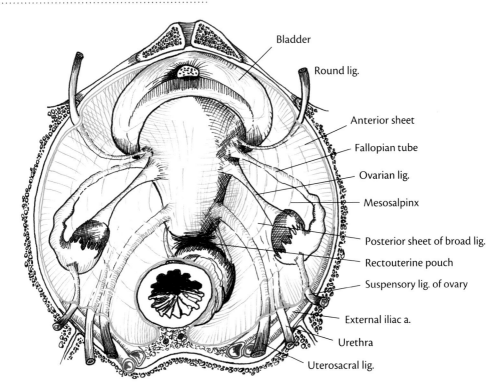

The broad ligament has thus formed the shape of a transverse quadrilateral septum which is acutely inclined in a forward and downward direction, with a markedly concave configuration oriented posteriorly (Fig. 2-26).

Distinction is usually made between two different parts:

- the inferior part, which is thick, immobile, and tightly associated with both the wall of the pelvis and the cervicoisthmic region of the uterus, as well as the vagina. It corresponds to the parametrium supporting the uterus and to the paravagina, the superior vaginal support
- the superior part or mesometrium, which includes three different parts:
  — the mesosalpinx
  — a funicular part called the round ligament
  — the mesovarium, which is supported by the ovarian ligament and the supensory ligament of the ovary

Umbilical fascia

This attaches to the vascular tentoria of the umbilical and vesical arteries, which it supports laterally from the median line. It is also attached to the median umbilical ligament (Fig. 2-27).

Fig. 2-26 Broad Ligament

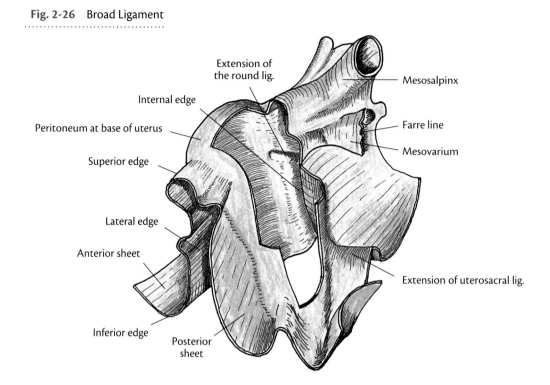

Extension of
the round lig.

Mesosalpinx

Internal edge

Farre line

Peritoneum at base of uterus

Mesovarium

Superior edge

Lateral edge

Anterior sheet

Extension of uterosacral lig.

Inferior edge

Posterior
sheet

Fig. 2-27 Umbilical Fascia

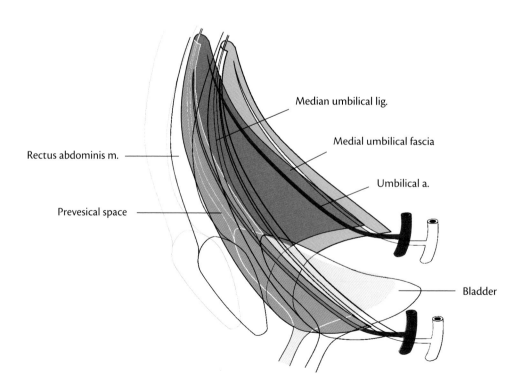

Median umbilical lig.

Medial umbilical fascia

Rectus abdominis m.

Umbilical a.

Prevesical space

Bladder

It is triangular in shape and markedly concave towards the back. It is attached to the umbilicus at its top and travels a short way posteriorly and inferiorly to reach the top of the bladder. On its arrival at the bladder, it suddenly broadens and folds back on itself to form a sulcus, which is concave posteriorly. This touches the anterior and lateral surfaces of the bladder and then descends along its surfaces until it reaches the floor of the pelvis where it terminates in the following manner:

- on the median line, it fuses with the pubovesical ligaments
- laterally, it joins with the pelvic aponeurosis of the pubovesical ligaments as far as the anterior edge of the two sciatic notches

The lateral edges of the umbilical ligament extend obliquely from the greater sciatic notches to the umbilicus. They are attached to the abdominopelvic wall at several points:

- at the bottom, to the aponeurosis of the internal obturator
- at the top, to the sheath of the transversalis fascia up to three or four centimeters below the arcuate line of the sheath of the rectus abdominis muscle

The inferior part of the umbilical ligament creates a retropubic space (also known as the Retzius space) between the bladder and the abdominal wall.

Sacrogenital folds

These structures, also known as the sacrorectogenitopubic membranes of Delbet, correspond to the tentoria of the internal iliac arteries. The membranes extend in a sagittal direction from behind and inside the sacral foramina as far as the posterior surface of the pubic bone anteriorly. They travel along the lateral borders of the pelvic viscera, towards which they extend fibers. On their medial surfaces, they are doubled up and reinforced by a nervous lamella corresponding to the hypogastric plexus (Fig. 2-28).

Summary of the Fasciae of the Perineum and Pelvis

There are three fasciae in the perineum which close the inferior part of the abdomen. These three fasciae are reinforced by the muscle systems that they invest.

The anterior peritoneum contains:

- the superficial fascia of the perineum, which joins the following fascial elements:
  - the superficial abdominal fasciae
  - the fasciae of the lower limbs
  - the aponeuroses of the gluteal muscles

- the middle fascia of the perineum, which is composed of two separate layers and which joins the following fascial elements:
  - the superficial fascia of the perineum
  - the deep perineal fascia
  - the deep abdominal fasciae
- the deep perineal fascia, an extremely strong tissue which invests the entire peritoneum and joins the following fascial elements:
  - the bottom of the middle fasciae of the perineum
  - the deep abdominal fasciae and the umbilical fascia
  - laterally, the aponeurosis of the internal obturator, which links it to the outside
  - the aponeurosis of the coccygeal muscle and, at a posterolateral point, the aponeurosis of the piriformis muscle; these two aponeuroses make up part of the deep perineal fascial system. Through its connection with the piriformis, this fascia establishes another link with the outside.
  - the presacral septum posteriorly
  - the entire periphery of the transversalis fascia

Above these fascial elements, and often derived from them, are:

- two central anteroposterior structures: the sacrogenital folds. These form compartments in a sagittal orientation with several septa which run from front to back:
- the umbilical ligament
- the vesicovaginal septum (in females)
- the rectovaginal septum (in females) and the rectovesical septum (in males)
- the presacral septum

The top of this region is formed by the peritoneum in males, and by a combination of the peritoneum and the parametrium in females.

A particular structure in this region warrants special attention: the central tendon of the perineum. This fibrous structure is located between the anus and the root of the scrotum in males, and between the rectum and the inferior root of the labia majora in females. It represents the lowermost point of the perineum and, by extension, of the entire thoracoabdominal cavity. It is formed by extensions of all three of the fascial elements of the perineum together with all the perineal muscles, apart from the ischiocavernosus and coccygeal muscles. Therefore, it represents the 'thread' which is used to close the bottom of the thoracoabdominal cavity.

Fig. 2-28 Sacrogenital folds

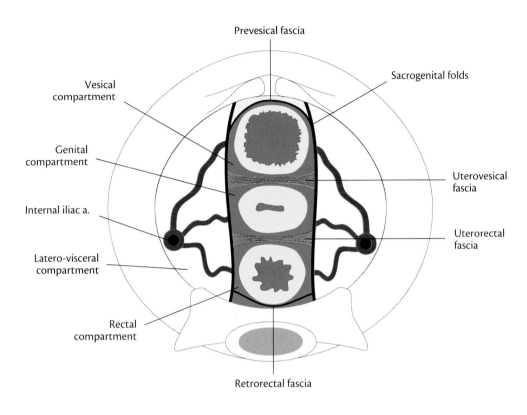

Table 2-7 Connections of the Perineal Fasciae

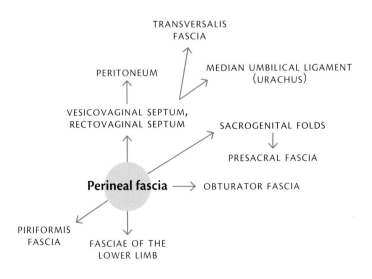

Fasciae of the Central Axis

INTERPTERYGOID FASCIA

This quadrilateral fascia is attached:

- on top, going from the back to the front
  - to the two lips of the petrotympanic fissure (also known as the glasserian fissure)
  - to the process of the petrous part of the temporal bone lying between the petrotympanic and tympanomastoid fissures
  - to the process of the sphenoid bone
  - to the medial edge of the foramen ovale
- on the bottom
  - to the maxilla immediately above the insertion of the medial pterygoid and also on the lingula of the mandible
- Its posterior edge is free.
- Its anterior edge:
  - is attached to the posterior edge of the lateral wing of the pterygoid fascia
  - lower down, it extends towards the lateral side of the base of the tongue where it joins the anterior extension of the buccinator fascia

The interpterygoid fascia is not uniform all over:

- its posterior portion is thick and strong and is also known as the sphenomandibular ligament
- its anterior portion is itself divided in two by the pterygomandibular raphe

PTERYGOTEMPOROMAXILLARY FASCIA

Located outside the interpterygoid fascia, it is inserted (Fig. 2-29):

- at the top into the greater wing of the sphenoid bone
- at the front to the superior part of the medial pterygoid wing
- its superior edge becomes free and thickens below and outside the foramen ovale to form the recessus epitympanicus
- at the bottom its insertion is continuous with the interpterygoid fascia

PALATINE APONEUROSIS

The palatine aponeurosis is an extremely strong fibrous membrane which invests the two veli palatini muscles and helps shape the soft palate. It is continuous with the palatine arch and occupies the anterior half of the soft palate for which it provides the skeletal framework. It is attached:

Fig. 2-29 Parasagittal Section through the Pharynx, Eustachian Tube and the Pterygoid Muscle

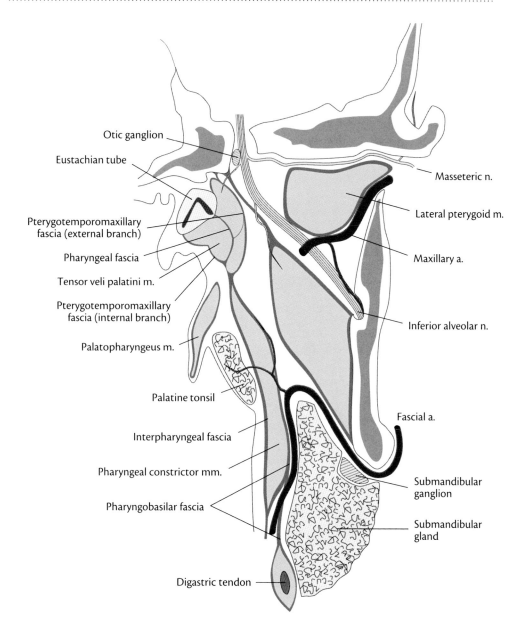

- at the front to the posterior edge of the palatine arch
- on the sides to the lower edge and to the hook of the medial wing of the pterygoid process
- at the back, it disappears into the thickness of the soft palate

It mainly consists of the tendinous fibers of the veli palatini muscles, with which it is continuous at the back.

The veli palatini muscles are continuous with the fasciae of the pharynx, which send out extensions to invest the descending portions of the tensor and levator veli palatini muscles.

PHARYNGOBASILAR AND BUCCOPHARYNGEAL FASCIAE

The pharyngobasilar fascia is a strong, fibrous membrane which covers the esophagus and the trachea. It continues up into the maxillopharyngeal space, investing the walls of the pharynx and extending down into the mediastinum. Above the superior constrictor of pharynx muscle, it joins the buccinator fascia and both are attached to the base of the cranium:

- on the basilar side of the occipital bone at the pharyngeal process
- on the inner side of the petrous part of the temporal bone anterior to and within the carotid foramen
- on the fibrous plate which covers the anterior lacerate foramen
- on the posterior, lateral part of the base of the pterygoid process
- on the lower, fibrous wall of the auditory tube
- on the pterygomaxillary ligament

Anteriorly, an outgrowth extends out following the course of the palatoglossus muscle up to the tongue. From the pharyngobasilar and buccinopharyngeal fasciae project extensions which cover the descending parts of the tensor and levator veli palatini muscles of the soft palate. Below the tensor veli palatini, the pharyngobasilar fascia is reinforced by the pterygomandibular raphe.

When it reaches the posterior edge of the thyroid, the pharyngobasilar fascia folds back on itself to form two sheets (Fig. 2-30):

- the deeper or internal sheet is continuous with the visceral portion and covers the trachea and the larynx as well as forming the thyrolaryngeal fascia
- the external sheet extends—from inside to outside—over the posterior side of the lateral lobe of the thyroid gland and, at the external limit on this side, joins with the deep sheet of the middle fascia, which completes the investment of the thyroid gland in front

From the anterior part of the visceral portion, along the inferior edge of the thyroid gland, a detachment extends outs which follows the course of the major thyroid veins, encloses the left brachiocephalic venous trunk, and continues as far as the pericardium. This extension is called the thyropericardial or cervicopericardial lamina (Rouviére).

Together, the cervicopericardial lamina, the adjacent part of the pericardium, the deep sheet of the middle fascia, and the superior sternopericardial ligament define a compartment which is occupied by the thymus (Fig. 2-31).

In the neck, there are sagittal extensions of the fascia or septa which attach it to the deep cervical fascia and thereby to the anterior processes of transversal fasciae. It is joined via a posterior extension to the styloid fascia to form the stylopharyngeal fascia. It is also attached to the greater and lesser horns of the hyoid

Fig. 2-30 Fasciae of the Neck: Sagittal Section

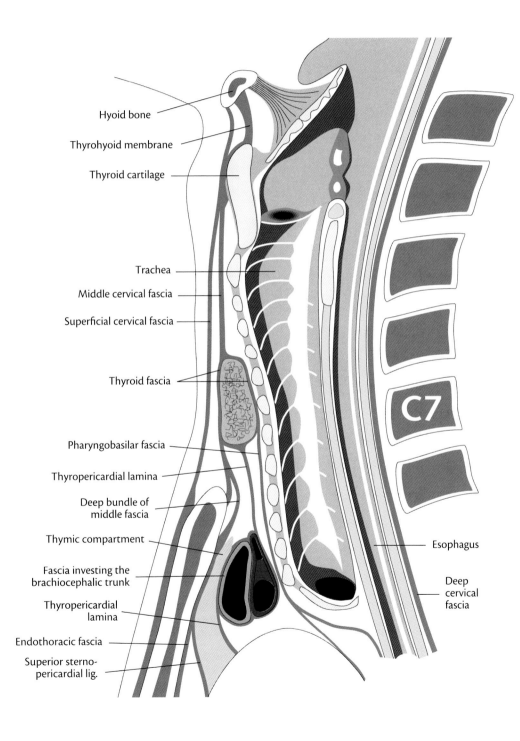

Hyoid bone

Thyrohyoid membrane

Thyroid cartilage

Trachea

Middle cervical fascia

Superficial cervical fascia

Thyroid fascia

Pharyngobasilar fascia

Thyropericardial lamina

Deep bundle of middle fascia

Thymic compartment

Fascia investing the brachiocephalic trunk

Thyropericardial lamina

Endothoracic fascia

Superior sterno-pericardial lig.

C7

Esophagus

Deep cervical fascia

bone. At the level of the superior constrictor of pharynx muscle, it extends into the pharynx to form an intrapharyngeal fascia. Its form is that of an incomplete cylinder because it only invests the posterior and lateral walls of the pharynx. Fibrous and strong at the top, it is thinner and more cellular lower down. It is continuous with the cellular lining of the esophagus at the back and with the pericardium in front.

Fig. 2-31 Thymic Compartment

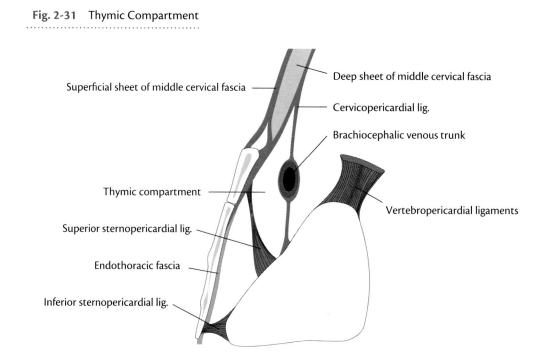

Table 2-8 Connections of the Pharyngobasilar Fascia

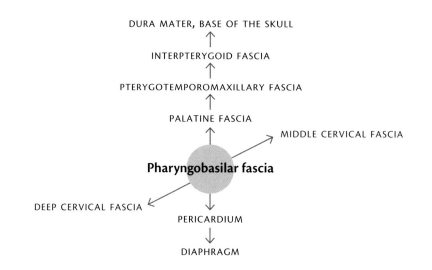

PERICARDIUM

The pericardium is the fibroserous sac that surrounds the heart. It consists of two different layers (Fig. 2-32):

- an internal, serous layer, comprised of two separate sheets:
  —a visceral sheet molded around the heart and the various vessels
  —another parietal sheet which covers the former
- an external, fibrous layer which hermetically seals the parietal sheet inside and serves both to protect and immobilize the heart

We will focus mainly on the fibrous pericardium, dealing briefly afterwards with the serous pericardium.

Fig. 2-32 Pericardium

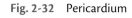

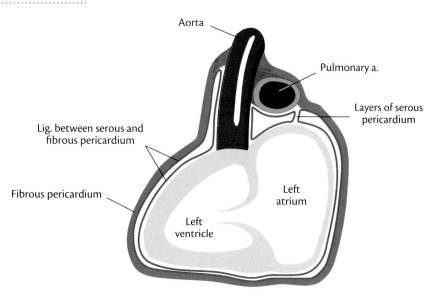

Fibrous Pericardium

As previously noted, the fibrous pericardium is continuous with the buccopharyngeal fascia.

The fibrous pericardium is a thick, strong membrane which covers the parietal layer of the serous pericardium, forming a fibrous sac which is crossed by the major vessels of the heart. Strong ligaments attach it to the diaphragm, the anterior and posterior walls of the thorax, as well as to structures of the neck.

Fibrous sac

The fibrous sac has a pearly white appearance and is composed of interlacing, curved fibers that are oriented in all directions. These condense into bands which form fibrous rings around the various vessels. Its shape is like that of a cone which has been truncated at the base, and it invests the heart. Its base lies on the diaphragm, more specifically on both the anterior leaflet of the central tendon and the anterior part of the left leaflet. However, it is separated from the diaphragm by a thin sheet of cellular adipose tissue which is continuous with the endothoracic fascia. This is called the phrenopericardial ligament.

Its anterior surface is adjacent to the anterior edge of the lungs, the anterior recess of the pleura, and the sternocostal cartilages. Its posterior surface is adjacent to the organs of the posterior mediastinum, especially the thoracic esophagus. The truncated tip tapers off into the vessels at the base of the heart above the serous pericardium and is, as has already been mentioned, continuous with the buccopharyngeal fascia.

The pericardium sends out a large number of extensions which form the ligaments for its attachment (Fig. 2-33).

Phrenopericardial ligaments

These three ligaments are the strongest of all and are continuous with the endothoracic fascia:

- the anterior ligament is attached to the anterior leaflet
- the right ligament is attached to the inferior vena cava
- the left is located to the left of the inferior vena cava

The latter two fit tightly around the inferior vena cava.

Sternopericardial ligaments

The superior sternopericardial ligament joins the manubrium of the sternum to the pericardium. This is an extension of the deep layer of the middle cervical fascia and is also continuous with the anterior wall of the visceral sheath of the neck. The inferior sternopericardial ligament joins the lower base of the xiphoid process to the pericardium.

Vertebropericardial ligaments

These are fibrous bands developed in the thickness of the sagittal septa. Their insertions are continuous with those of the sagittal septa of the buccinator fascia on the prevertebral fascia as of the sixth cervical vertebra. Up to the third thoracic vertebra, they terminate at the bottom at the upper part of the pericardium.

Cervicopericardial ligaments

The cervicopericardial ligaments form what is known as the thyropericardial lamina of Richet, an extension of the visceral sheath of the neck. This detaches at the sheath of the thyroid gland, forms a frontal lamina which defines the thymic compartment, and terminates at the anterior surface of the pericardium.

Visceropericardial ligaments

These are simple auxiliary fibrous tracts which join the pericardium:

- posteriorly to the thoracic esophagus: these are known as the esophagopericardial ligaments
- superiorly to the tracheal bifurcation: these are known as tracheopericardial and bronchopericardial ligaments
- laterally to the pulmonary veins to form the alae of the pericardium

Fig. 2-33   Pericardial Ligaments

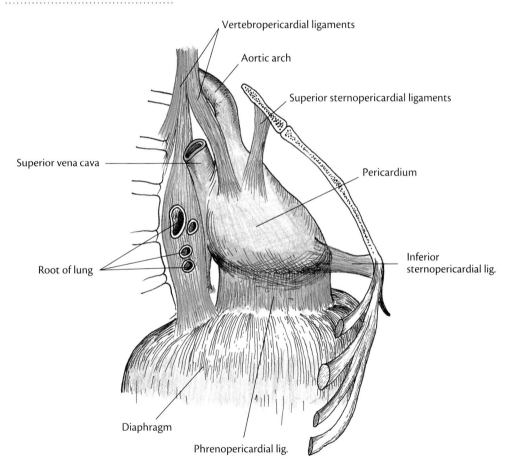

Vertebropericardial ligaments

Aortic arch

Superior sternopericardial ligaments

Superior vena cava

Pericardium

Root of lung

Inferior sternopericardial lig.

Diaphragm

Phrenopericardial lig.

Serous Pericardium

The serous pericardium consists of two different layers:

- the visceral layer, which is molded around the heart
- the parietal sheet, which invests the visceral sheet and is intimately associated with the fibrous pericardium

These two layers fold back on themselves to demarcate a sealed space around the major vessels.

The fibrous pericardium is inelastic and is innervated by the phrenic nerve. The serous pericardium receives vasomotor and sensory nerve fibers coming from the coronary plexus. Stimulation of these nerves does not induce any kind of pain.

Table 2-9   Connections of the Pericardium

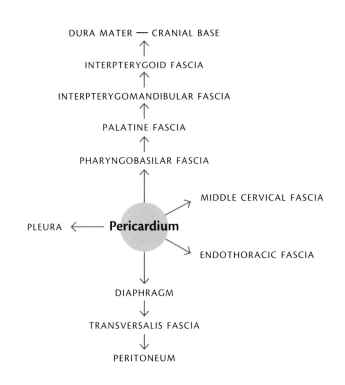

DURA MATER — CRANIAL BASE
↑
INTERPTERYGOID FASCIA
↑
INTERPTERYGOMANDIBULAR FASCIA
↑
PALATINE FASCIA
↑
PHARYNGOBASILAR FASCIA
↑
                              → MIDDLE CERVICAL FASCIA
PLEURA ← — **Pericardium**
                              ↘ ENDOTHORACIC FASCIA
↓
DIAPHRAGM
↓
TRANSVERSALIS FASCIA
↓
PERITONEUM

Summary of the Central Fascial Axis

The central fascial axis is composed of:

- interpterygoid and pterygotemporomaxillary fasciae, and the palatine aponeurosis, which anchor it at the base of the skull. It continues into the:
- pharyngobasilar and buccopharyngeal fasciae, which is itself continuous with the pericardium

This axis is continuous:

- superiorly with the meninges via the cranial nerves

- around its edges and going inferiorly from the top:
  - posteriorly with the deep cervical fascia via the sagittal membranes and with the endothoracic fascia anteriorly and the pericardial ligaments posteriorly
  - anteriorly with the middle cervical fascia, together with which it constitutes the sheath of the thyroid gland and the thymic cavity
  - laterally with the pleura at the level of the thorax
- inferiorly with the diaphragm

Diaphragm

The diaphragm is the main muscle involved in breathing, yet aside from this role, it can also be considered as an important fascial element. The central tendon is fibrous. It descends from the transverse septum that originates in the cervical area of the embryo and therefore brings with it the entire fascial column which we have been discussing.

The diaphragm forms a connection between the thoracic and abdominal fascial systems at the same time as it separates these two major body cavities (Fig. 2-34). Its upper part is covered by the endothoracic fascia doubled up with the pleura. This fascia extends down into the abdomen in the form of the transversalis fascia. Its inferior surface is lined by the peritoneum, and the renal fasciae project from this area. It is also attached to the fasciae associated with the psoas muscle.

The peritoneum also serves to attach the liver and the stomach to the diaphragm. At its superior surface, it is itself suspended by a fascial sheath formed by the pericardium, the buccopharyngeal fascia, and then the interpterygoid fascia and the palatine aponeurosis. This fixes everything to the base of the skull.

In the anteroposterior direction, this sheath is stabilized by the vertebropericardial and sternopericardial ligaments.

The diaphragm represents a continuation between the fasciae of the base of the skull, the neck, and the thorax, and those of the abdomen. It is a relay point and an important shock absorber, as will be discussed in detail in Chapter 6 below.

Internal Thoracoabdominal Fasciae

PLEURA

There are two pleurae, one right and one left, entirely distinct from one another.

Fig. 2-34   Links between Thorax, Abdomen and Kidneys

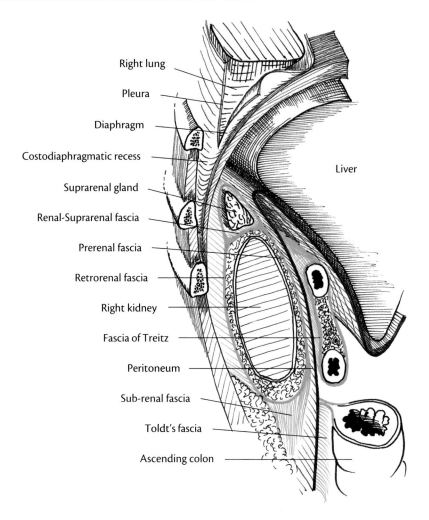

Right lung
Pleura
Diaphragm
Costodiaphragmatic recess
Suprarenal gland
Renal-Suprarenal fascia
Prerenal fascia
Retrorenal fascia
Right kidney
Fascia of Treitz
Peritoneum
Sub-renal fascia
Toldt's fascia
Ascending colon

Liver

They are serous membranes composed of two layers:

- a visceral layer, which invests the lung
- a parietal layer, which lines the walls of the thoracic cavity

The parietal and visceral layers are continuous with one another at the hilum of the lung, where the pleura fold back on themselves.

Between the two layers there is a virtual, fluid-filled cavity, the pleural cavity.

Visceral Pleura

The visceral pleura covers the whole surface of the lung except for an area on its mediastinal side at the hilum, where it folds back to form the parietal pleura. The fold line continues on below the hilum in order to form the pulmonary ligament.

The visceral pleura penetrates within the lung to line the pulmonary fissures, after which it splits to cover the various lobes of the lung (Fig. 2-35).

The visceral pleura is joined to the pulmonary parenchyma via a thin layer of subpleural cellular tissue which continues into the parenchyma to form the framework of the lung, or pulmonary interstitium.

Fig. 2-35 Anterior Borders of the Pleura and Lungs

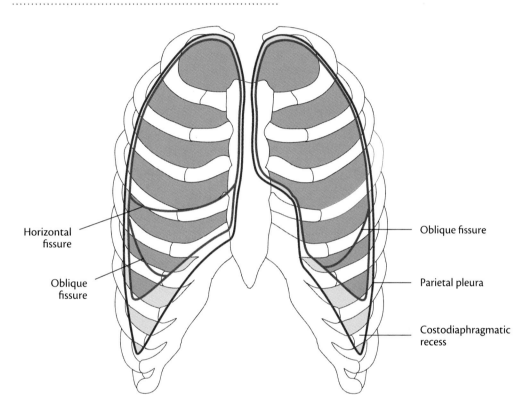

Parietal Pleura

The parietal pleura lines almost all of the deep surface of the thoracic cavity. It is innervated by the intercostal, thoracoabdominal, and phrenic nerves. It joins the wall via the endothoracic fascia, which it then divides on the inside. Distinction is usually made between different segments of the pleura:

- a costal segment, or the costal pleura
- a mediastinal segment, or the mediastinal pleura
- a diaphragmatic segment, or the diaphragmatic pleura

These three elements continue independently to form the pleural pouches.

Costal pleura

This segment lines the deep surface of the ribs and the intercostal spaces from which it is separated by the endothoracic fascia.

- Anteriorly, it extends as far as the edges of the sternum and then folds back posteriorly to form the mediastinal pleura.
- Inferiorly, it folds back to form the diaphragmatic pleura

Diaphragmatic pleura

Thinner than the costal pleura, this segment is attached to the endothoracic fascia and thus to the superior surface of the cupulae of the diaphragm, strongly but incompletely. On the left, it leaves a portion of the diaphragm free for insertion of the pericardium. On the right, it covers the entire part of the cupula outside an anteroposterior line which passes along the lateral edge of the opening for the inferior vena cava.

Mediastinal pleura

The mediastinal pleura covers all the mediastinal structures in an anteroposterior direction, from the sternum at the front as far as the costovertebral sulcus at the back. These structures are:

- in the anterior mediastinum: the pericardium, the phrenic nerve and accompanying vessels, the thymus, the right brachiocephalic trunk, and the superior and inferior vena cava
- in the posterior mediastinum: the trachea, the esophagus, the azygos vein, the right vagus nerve on the right, the descending thoracic aorta, the hemiazygos vein, and, at the top, the thoracic duct on the left

At the root of the lung, the mediastinal pleura forms a quasi-circular sleeve around the components of the root, lining its anterior, posterior, and superior surfaces. On the outside, around the hilum, it folds back to form the visceral pleura. The folding of the pleura near the hilum continues into the diaphragm via the triangularly-shaped pulmonary ligament.

The ligament of the left lung is more or less vertical, whereas that of the right lung forms an oblique angle at the bottom and behind, where it is distorted by the inferior vena cava.

On the inside, each of the pulmonary ligaments meets the lateral edge of the esophagus via the esophageal fascia, to which they are strongly attached.

Pleural dome

A pleural dome tops each lung. It is strongly attached to the endothoracic fascia, which thickens significantly in order to constitute the cervicothoracic diaphragm. Within this diaphragm, the following ligaments which suspend the pleura can be distinguished (Fig. 2-36):

- the costopleural ligament
- the transverse cupular ligament
- the pleurovertebral ligament

Fig. 2-36   Pleural Dome

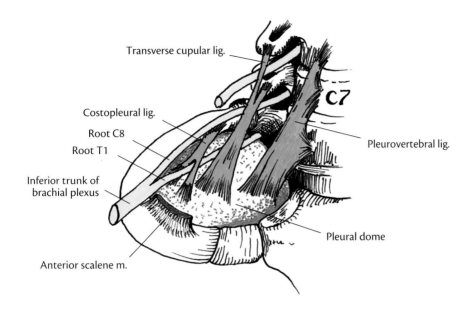

Transverse cupular lig.

C7

Costopleural lig.

Root C8

Root T1

Pleurovertebral lig.

Inferior trunk of
brachial plexus

Pleural dome

Anterior scalene m.

Summary of the Pleurae

The pleura consists of two layers separated by a virtual space which is lubricated to allow the layers to slide against one another.

- The inner layer, or visceral pleura, invests the lung and splits deep down
  to form the fissures of the lung and invest the various lobes and lobules.

- The outer layer, or parietal pleura, anchors the lung to external
  structures and allows it to function as a pump

It joins:

- on the inside, the pericardium

- around its edge, the endothoracic fascia, and thereby the inner thoracic
  wall

- at the bottom, the diaphragm

- at the top, the endothoracic fascia ,and thereby the cervical fasciae via
  the suspensory ligaments of the pleura

Table 2-10 Connections of the Pleura

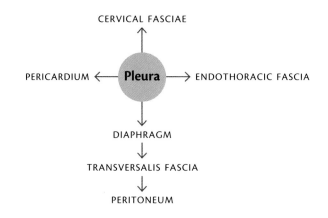

PERITONEUM AND PERITONEAL CAVITY

The peritoneum is a serous membrane which lines the deep surface of the abdominal cavity, the pelvic cavity, and all the organs therein. The peritoneum undergoes multiple changes at various stages of embryonic and fetal development until, in the adult, it is extensively folded back on itself, creating a highly complex surface which is explained by embryology (Fig. 2-37).

As is the case with all serous membranes, it consists of two layers:

- a parietal layer lining the deep surface of the abdominal cavit
- a visceral layer covering the superficial surface of the abdominal viscera

These two layers define a virtual cavity, namely, the peritoneal cavity with the lowest point being Douglas' pouch—this is the rectouterine pouch in females and the rectovesical pouch in males. The peritoneal cavity can be represented as basically a closed sac which contains all the abdominal organs and other viscera. It should be noted, however, that the peritoneum is not hermetically sealed in the female because there is an opening at the level of the ovary called the Farre line. This discontinuity allows the peritoneal fluid to flow across the fallopian tubes and also accounts for why ascending peritoneal infections of gynecological origin are possible in women.

In males, when the testes descend, the peritoneum forms an invagination like the finger of a glove at the level of the testes (the tunica vaginalis testis), which takes with it the transversalis fascia (a tunica fibrosa) and fibers of the transversalis and cremaster muscles.

The parietal peritoneum is often separated from the abdominal wall by subperitoneal tissue. While abundant and loose at the lower part of the wall where the peritoneum is easily detached, everywhere else it is relatively sparse, tight, and solidly attaches the peritoneum to the wall of the cavity.

Fig. 2-37   The Male Peritoneum

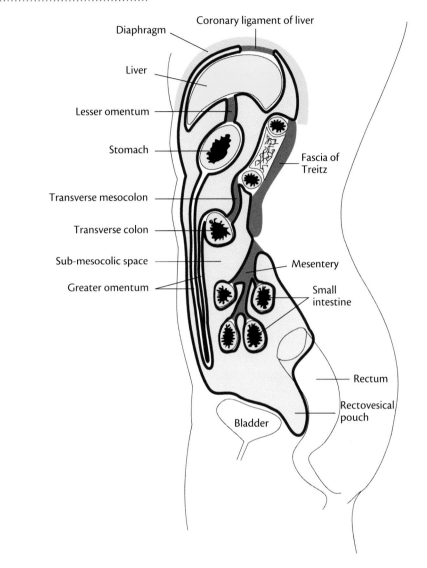

Parietal Peritoneum

The parietal peritoneum lines the deep surface of the abdominal cavity.
Distinction is made among:

- the diaphragmatic parietal peritoneum
- the posterior parietal peritoneum
- the anterior parietal peritoneum
- the inferior or pelvic parietal peritoneum

Diaphragmatic parietal peritoneum

This is strongly attached to the inferior surface of the diaphragm, except at the
level of the coronary ligament of the liver anteriorly, as will be explained later.

Posterior parietal peritoneum

This lines the transversalis fascia and thereby the posterior wall of the abdominal cavity. However, it is separated from the abdominal wall by the retroperitoneal space which contains:

- in the center, the large prevertebral vessels (the aorta and the vena cava)
- laterally, the kidneys, the suprarenal glands, and the ureters

The ureter is attached to the peritoneum anteriorly via its connective tissue sheath formed by the subperitoneal fascia. The ureter moves with the peritoneum unless it becomes detached.

Anterior parietal peritoneum

This lines the deep surface of the anterolateral wall of the abdominal cavity from which it is separated by a subperitoneal cellular space. This space gradually narrows as it continues forwards towards the median line.

In its subumbilical part, it steadily recedes from the wall, inhibited from behind by the umbilicoprevesical aponeurosis. Here, the perineum is lifted by the median umbilical ligament and the medial umbilical ligaments, which go on to form three fossae:

- the internal inguinal fossa
- the medial inguinal fossa
- the lateral inguinal fossa

The lateral fossa constitutes the medial opening of the inguinal canal through which the spermatic cord passes. These fossae correspond to weak points in the abdominal wall through which a loop of intestine can be forced, creating an inguinal hernia. Just above the inguinal ligament, the anterior parietal peritoneum is separated from the parietal plane by a cellular space called the retroinguinal space, or Bogros space.

Pelvic parietal peritoneum

The pelvic parietal peritoneum lines the walls of the pelvic cavity and, on the sides and the median line, covers the subperitoneal space and all the viscera it contains (namely, from back to front, the rectum, the internal genital organs, and the bladder).

It covers the lateral and superior surfaces of the bladder, to which it is strongly attached. Behind the bladder:

- in males, it covers the base of the seminal vesicles, forms the rectovesical pouch, and goes on to cover the rectum, behind which it forms the pararectal fossa on each side;
- in females, it is strongly attached to the parametrium, which covers the uterus and its accessories, and forms two structures:

    —the anterior, relatively shallow vesicouterine pouch

    —the posterior, rectouterine pouch

It should be remembered that these structures can be a focus for both collection of fluids (especially the lower rectouterine pouch) as well as trapping of intestinal loops.

Visceral Peritoneum

This lines the deep surface of the parietal peritoneum and the superficial surface of the abdominal viscera. It is strongly attached. The peritoneal layers define the peritoneal cavity, which is occupied by the viscera of the digestive tract. This cavity is divided by a number of different folds which create septa, fossae, and recesses. The largest of these recesses is the posterior cavity of the omenta, which divides the peritoneal cavity into two parts:

- the greater peritoneal sac
- the lesser peritoneal sac, known as the omental bursa

Another important fold of the peritoneum links the transverse colon to the posterior wall and forms an oblique septum at the bottom and at the front, which divides the greater peritoneal cavity into two different compartments. These are known as the supracolic and infracolic compartments, or the superior and inferior compartments of the abdomen.

Next we will concentrate on the peritoneal folds. Their organization is highly complex and, in order to gain a better understanding, it is worth returning to their embryology.

Peritoneal Folds

The peritoneal serous membrane is highly complex because of a large number of different types of folds which are referred to as:

- mesentery
- ligaments
- omenta

Mesentery

The mesentery attach the abdominal viscera to the peritoneal wall and provide them with their blood supply and innervation. A mesentery is formed whenever the parietal peritoneum covering an organ folds back upon itself to invest the organ and the nerves and vessels supplying it. The parietal area circumscribed by these two layers represent the insertion root of the mesentery. The length of the mesentery affords each organ a certain degree of mobility within the peritoneal cavity.

In the primary embryological arrangement, the following can be distinguished:

- a mesogastrium at the level of the stomach
- a mesentery at the level of the small intestine
- a mesocolon at the level of the large intestine

By virtue of the lengthening of the primitive intestine and gastric and intestinal rotation, certain organs are pressed up against the posterior abdominal wall. The posterior layer of the mesothelium fuses with the posterior parietal peritoneum. The fasciae essentially become avascular cleavage planes which are associated more or less strongly with the walls of the organs that they invest.

After birth, the terminal part of the esophagus, the entire initial part of the stomach, and the left end of the pancreas, are coupled through the posterior mesogastrium with:

- the duodenopancreas, which is itself linked through Treitz's fascia
- the ascending and descending colon are linked through Toldt's fascia

The stomach, the first part of the duodenum, the small intestine, the transverse colon, and the sigmoid colon remain mobile and are joined to the wall by mesenteries.

Mesenteries

The connecting fasciae that make up the mesenteries are derived from the mesothelia (Fig. 2-38).

▶ MESENTERIES OF THE STOMACH

These two mesenteries are constituted by the falx-like folds of peritoneum that enclose vascular bundles. The first is the gastropancreatic fold, which extends

Fig. 2-38   Omenta and Mesentery
of Stomach

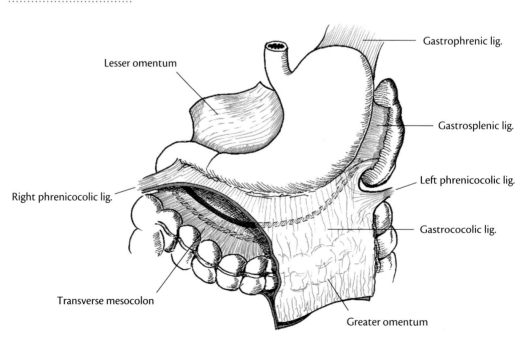

Gastrophrenic lig.

Lesser omentum

Gastrosplenic lig.

Left phrenicocolic lig.

Right phrenicocolic lig.

Gastrocolic lig.

Transverse mesocolon

Greater omentum

from the celiac trunk at the upper third of the lesser curvature. Its lower edge, concave at the bottom and oriented to the front and right, delineates the omental foramen at the top, giving access at the back to the cavity of the omenta. It encases the hepatic and left gastric arteries.

The hepatic fold is also known as the duodenopancreatic ligament. It is oriented in the opposite direction with its superior edge free and concave at the top, defining the lower part of the foramen.

▶ MESENTERY OF THE SMALL INTESTINE

The mesentery of the jejunoileum , usually simply referred to as the mesentery, is attached to the posterior wall of the abdomen and provides the blood supply and innervation to the bulk of the small intestine. It is in the shape of a segment of a circle. It consists of two parts: the root, which is immobile and very strongly attached to the posterior abdominal wall, especially at its middle segment; and the intestinal border, which is highly mobile as it connects to the edge of the intestines which are five to six meters in length.

About fifteen centimeters in length and eighteen millimeters in diameter, the root of the mesentery draws an oblique broken line that goes inferiorly and to the right from the duodenojejunal junction. Distinction is usually made between three different segments:

- The superior segment travels obliquely inferiorly and to the right. It extends from the duodenojejunal junction, where it is strongly attached to the left transverse process of the second lumbar vertebra by the muscle of Treitz, and to the lower edge of the third part of the duodenum, anterior to the body of L3.
- The shorter middle vertical segment represents the most solidly fixed element and it is here that the superior mesenteric vessels penetrate the mesentery. It projects onto L3 and L4.
- The inferior segment becomes oblique again, traveling inferiorly and to the right. It extends from the L4/L5 disk to the ileocecal junction above the right common iliac artery, crossing the ureter and the spermatic (or ovarian) vessels.

▶ TRANSVERSE MESOCOLON

This forms a transverse lamina stretching from the right abdominal wall to the left wall.

Obliquely running inferiorly and anteriorly, it divides the peritoneal cavity into the superior (supracolic) and inferior (infracolic) compartments. It attaches the transverse colon to the posterior wall. Its anterior edge is very loose, especially on the left, and the posterior edge is attached to the posterior wall. It crosses the head of the pancreas, to which it attaches. Then it passes from the duodenojejunal junction along the lower edge of the body of the pancreas. Its left part goes on to form the lower wall of the posterior cavity of the omenta (Fig. 2-39).

Fig. 2-39   Fasciae of the Pancreas and Duodenum

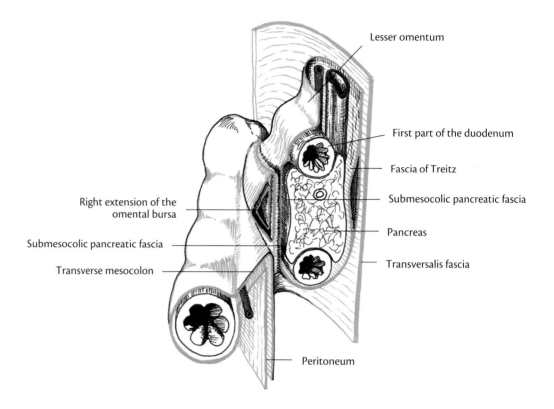

SIGMOID MESOCOLON

The sigmoid colon is attached to the posterior wall by a two-rooted meso-colon:

- The primary root descends vertically and in the medial direction, going from the inferior mesocolon to the anterior face of S3.
- The secondary root runs obliquely inferiorly and to the left, going from the inferior mesocolon to the medial edge of the left psoas along the lateral edge of the common iliac and external iliac arteries, finally crossing the spermatic (or ovarian) vessels and the ureter.

The mesocolon often sends out extensions, which anchor the sigmoid colon to the wall and to the neighboring organs. These include small ligaments which join the colon to the wall of the common iliac artery, thereby extending the secondary root towards the left, join the sigmoid mesocolon to the left fallopian tube, and stretch from the sigmoid mesocolon to the right layer of the mesentery.

Fasciae

As previously mentioned, these represent a joining of different mesenteries.

▶ TREITZ'S FASCIA

The fascia linking the duodenum and the head of the pancreas, it provides a solid anchor for these organs. It inserts at the junction between the second and third parts of the duodenum and extends to the transverse process of L2. The muscle of Treitz itself sends out an extension to the left pillar of the diaphragm at the right edge of the esophagus, which continues around the aortic opening.

▶ TOLDT'S FASCIA

Toldt's fascia is the fascia connecting the posterior wall of the ascending and descending colon.

For the ascending colon, it extends from the cecum to the right colic flexure. It attaches the colon to the posterior parietal peritoneum. However, in a few cases, there is no connection and therefore the colon is completely free in the abdominal cavity.

It continues downwards to merge into the ligaments which join the lateral edge of the cecum to the lumboiliac wall. The internal edge of the cecum is also joined to the iliac wall via the retrocolic ligament, which is no more than an extension of the lower insertion of the root of the mesentery. The root of the mesentery provides a point of attachment for the appendix, that is, the mesoappendix, which itself sends out an extension downwards in the form of the appendico-ovarian ligament.

The upper part of Toldt's fascia extends as far as the right colic flexure and forms its deep attachment plane. Here, the following can be distinguished: a renocolic ligament that attaches it to the kidneys, and a phrenicocolic ligament that attaches to the diaphragm.

It should also be remembered that other ligaments are associated with the right colic flexure:

- the middle plane with the cystoduodenocolic and hepatocolic ligaments
- the superficial plane with the omentocoloparietal ligament

For the descending colon, Toldt's fascia extends from the left colic flexure to the sigmoid colon. It attaches the colon to the posterior peritoneum and continues at the bottom into the sigmoid mesocolon. Its upper part forms the deep attachment plane for the left colic flexure.

It should also be remembered that other ligaments are associated with the left colic flexure:

- the middle plane with the splenocolic ligament, which extends down into the gastrosplenic and splenopancreatic ligaments
- the superficial plane (the larger) with the left phrenicocolic ligament, creating the bed for the spleen, whose base lies on its superior surface

It should be noted that the various segments of the colon detach easily from the posterior wall and that their peritoneal attachments tend to extend towards the center of the abdomen. This explains why it is much easier to bring them back towards the median line of the abdomen than it is to stretch them laterally.

Ligaments

The designation *peritoneal ligament* is given to peritoneal lamina having two layers which join visceral elements to one another or to the abdominal wall, and which do not contain any significant vascular plexus. Certain ones are derived by folding of the peritoneum and others are extensions of the mesenteries or the omenta. There are a great number of such ligaments. Some provide very strong attachment; others are inconstant and variable, and their role in stabilization is relatively minor.

▶ ROUND LIGAMENT OF THE LIVER

This is a remnant of the umbilical vein which runs within the free edge of a vast sagittal fold called the falciform or suspensory ligament. It creates a vertical, anteroposterior septum which goes from the umbilicus to the posterosuperior surface of the liver and joins the convex side of the liver to the diaphragm and the anterior wall of the abdominal cavity. It is composed of two layers joined at the anterior portion as far as the umbilicus, where it continues into the medial umbilical ligament (a remnant of the urachus).

Superiorly, at the level of the posterosuperior edge of the liver, the two layers separate: one carries on to the right over the right lobe of the liver while the other carries on to the left over the entire breadth of the left lobe, where it continues as the superior layer of the coronary ligament.

▶ CORONARY LIGAMENT

The coronary ligament joins the posterior side of the liver to the diaphragm. It consists of two layers:

- an anterosuperior layer, which folds back from the diaphragm to the liver along its posterosuperior edge. On the median line, it continues as the falciform ligament, as previously explained.
- an inferior layer, which folds back onto the vertical portion of the diaphragm, carries along its inferior edge and over the vena cava, and finally the transverse part of the ligamentum venosum (the remnants of the fetal ductus venosus) where it rejoins the posterior layer of the lesser omentum.

The coronary ligament sends out three extensions around the inferior vena cava:

- the inconstant mesohepatocaval extension, which extends around the inferior vena cava
- the right and left triangular ligaments, formed when the superior layer joins up with the inferior layer of the coronary ligament

These two ligaments terminate in a free edge which extends vertically from the diaphragm to the upper surface of the liver.

It should be remembered that, from an embryological point of view, the liver develops in the transverse septum (which constitutes the central tendon of the diaphragm), which is itself derived from the brachial arch.

Because of its increase in volume, it descends down into the abdominal cavity, stretching out its attachments to form the falciform, coronary ligament, and the lesser omentum. At the same time, it becomes surrounded by the fibrous capsule of the liver which comes from the central tendon. Subsequently, it is completely covered by the peritoneum, except for in the plane in which the coronary ligament is given off, where it is in direct contact with the diaphragm.

▶ GASTROPHRENIC LIGAMENT

This is found where the two layers of the gastric peritoneum fold back over the diaphragmatic peritoneum. It extends from the posterior side of the great tuberosity to the left leaflet of the diaphragm. It continues to the right as the high part of the lesser omentum, and to the left with the gastrosplenic ligament.

▶ GASTROCOLIC LIGAMENT

Derived from the greater omentum, this ligament extends from the greater curvature of the stomach down to the transverse colon.

▶ BROAD LIGAMENT

The broad ligament can be considered as attaching the peritoneum to the uterus and its accessories, as previously discussed.

▶ SUSPENSORY LIGAMENTS OF THE COLIC FLEXURES

These are the right and left parietocolic ligaments, lateral extensions of the greater omentum, which represent the most important attachments of the flexures of the colon.

Omenta

These are lamina of the peritoneum, some of which contain one or more vascular plexuses and connect to one or another of the organs located in the peritoneal cavity. There are four different omenta, three of which are attached to the stomach. Note that the last two described here are more commonly referred to as ligaments.

▶ LESSER OMENTUM

This quadrilateral lamina is also known as the gastrohepatic omentum. It is located in the frontal plane and extends from the lesser gastric curvature over the right edge of the esophagus and the first part of the duodenum to the interior surface of the liver close to the hilum. It then makes a right angle turn backwards to follow the fissure of the ligamentum venosum and the left vertical sulcus as far as the posterior surface of the liver before inserting into the diaphragm.

It should be remembered that the lesser omentum receives extensions of the coronary and the gastrophrenic ligaments. On the right, it leaves a free edge, which will constitute the epiploic foramen, to give access to the posterior omental fossa. In its mass are found the bile ducts and the vascular plexus of the liver.

▶ GREATER OMENTUM

This quadrilateral lamina is also known as the gastrocolic omentum. It invests the intestine at the front like a more or less extensive apron. Superiorly, it is attached to the stomach's greater curvature, forms the gastrocolic ligament, and then passes at the front from the transverse colon (to which it is attached) as it descends into the abdominal cavity. It terminates with a free edge.

Laterally, it sends out extensions to the abdominal wall which go on to form the suspensory ligaments of the colic flexures. The left edge of the gastrocolic ligament continues superiorly in the leftward direction with the gastrosplenic omentum. This is a broad peritoneal lamina which consists of four superimposed layers.

▶ GASTROSPLENIC OMENTUM

This is more commonly known as the gastrosplenic ligament. It is a superiorly directed continuation of the greater omentum. This two-layered lamina extends from the greater curvature of the stomach as far as the anterior side of the hilum of the spleen. Here, the two layers separate:

- the anterior layer goes on to line the anterior side of the medial surface of the spleen
- the posterior layer folds back on itself at the hilum to form the right anterior layer of the splenopancreatic omentum

▶ SPLENOPANCREATIC OMENTUM

Composed of two layers, the splenopancreatic omentum or ligament is inserted in front and behind at the level of the tail of the pancreas and in the posterior parietal plane. It extends as far as the hilum of the spleen. Its right anterior layer is continuous with the posterior layer of the splenogastric omentum. Its short posterior layer turns back to become the posterior parietal peritoneum.

▶ POSTERIOR OMENTAL FOSSA

The four omenta define an area to the rear of the stomach which is flattened in the anteroposterior direction—the posterior cavity of the omenta—which is demarcated:

- posteriorly by the posterior parietal peritoneum
- anteriorly by the lesser omentum, the posterior surface of the stomach, and the transverse colon

- inferiorly by the transverse mesocolon
- on the left, by the gastrosplenic and splenopancreatic omenta

This cavity communicates on the right with the greater peritoneal cavity via the epiploic foramen. The posterior cavity of the omenta provides a lubricated surface across which the stomach can slide and affords the stomach mobility within the abdominal cavity.

The main nerves supplying the peritoneum are the phrenic nerve, the thoracoabdominal nerves, and the sensory and vasomotor nerves coming from the lumbar plexus. The root of the mesentery contains pain nerves which are particularly sensitive to stretching distortions.

Summary of the Peritoneum

The peritoneum consists of two layers separated by a virtual space which allows them to slide with respect to one another.

Parietal peritoneum. Lines the deep surface of the abdominal cavity and connects:

- superiorly with the diaphragm
- laterally with the transversalis fascia
- inferiorly with the organs of the true pelvis and the perineum via the following septa:
    - the vesicorectal septum
    - the vesicovaginal septum
    - the rectovaginal septum
    - the prostatic septum

Visceral peritoneum. Does not make direct contact with the parietal peritoneum but is attached to it many times over via:

- ligaments
- mesenteries
- fasciae
- omenta,

which provide support for elements of the vascular and nervous systems and also invest all the abdominal organs.

- In males, the peritoneum extends into an invagination passing through the inguinal canal as far as the scrotum.
- In females, the peritoneum is not hermetically sealed and is in communication with the fallopian tubes via Farres lines.

Table 2-11 Connections of the Peritoneum

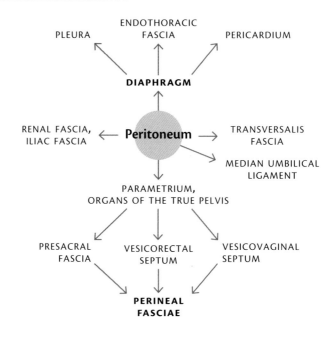

Meninges

The brain and the spinal cord are entirely enveloped by three concentric membranes, the meninges, which consist of (from the outside inwards):

- the dura mater
- the arachnoid membrane
- the pia mater

We will first deal with those in the cranium, and then in the spinal cord (Fig. 2-40)

DURA MATER

Cranial Dura Mater

The cranial dura mater is a thick (between 0.3 and 10 millimeters in thickness—thickest around the foramen magnum), fibrous membrane which is extremely strong. It is composed of bundles of connective tissue mixed with elastic fibers which line the internal surface of the cranial cavity and are so intimately associated with the periosteum that they are difficult to separate. The distinction between the periosteum and the dura mater is only very apparent at the foramen magnum, where they separate, and the dura mater continues downward to invest the spinal cord. According to recent research in dogs, the thickness of the dura mater varies according to the intracranial pressure: the higher the pressure, the thicker the membrane (Kuchiwaki, 1995). The outer and inner surfaces of the dura mater are distinct.

Fig. 2-40   Meninges and Cerebrospinal Fluid

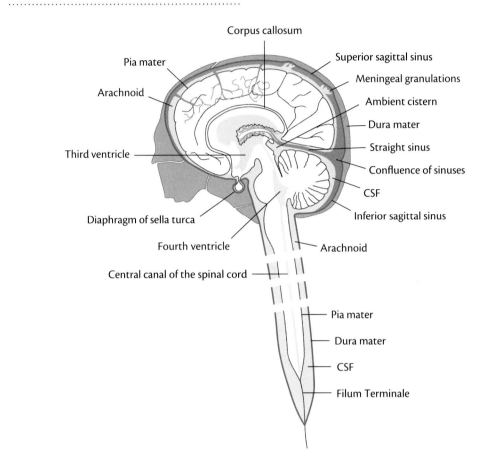

Outer surface

The outer surface of the dura mater of the brain lines the entire surface of the cranial cavity, attaching to the wall via fibrous vascular and nervous extensions. The mode of attachment differs in the vault and the base of the cranium.

▶ VAULT

Attachment is relatively weak, apart from at the sutures, where it is strong. It is relatively easy to detach, as reflected by the fact that Marchant named the following area the "detachable region":

- anteroposteriorly, from the posterior edges of the lesser wings of the sphenoid bone up to within two or three centimeters from the internal occipital protruberance
- superoinferiorly, from a few centimeters lateral to the falx cerebri to a horizontal line drawn between the posterior edge of the lesser wings

which touches the upper edge of the petrous portion of the temporal bone, and then passes above the horizontal portion of the lateral sinus

▶ BASE

Here the dura mater is very strongly attached to the periosteum, especially at the following points:

- the crista galli
- the posterior edges of the lesser wings of the sphenoid
- the posterior and anterior clinoid processes
- the upper edge of the petrous part of the temporal bone
- the rim of the foramen magnum

The strength of attachment of the dura mater varies with age, tending to be stronger in adults than in children and steadily increasing with advancing age, even in the normal as opposed to the disease state.

It invests all the vessels and nerves crossing the cranium with extensions that follow with them through their respective openings. Beyond the openings, they separate to continue into the extracranial periosteum. These extensions invest:

- the hypoglossal nerve as far as the anterior condylar fossa
- the vagus, glossopharyngeal, and spinal nerves, and the internal jugular vein as far as below the jugular foramen
- the facial and auditory nerve in the internal auditory tube, where it fuses with the periosteum
- the mandibular nerve in the foramen ovale
- the maxillary nerve in the foramen rotundum
- the olfactory fibers as far as the nasal fossae

In the optic canal and the superior orbital fissure, the dura mater continues into the orbit where it joins with the periosteum of this cavity. It also provides a fibrous sheath which goes as far as the eyeball where it is continuous with the sclera.

The dura mater forms a falciform fold above the optic nerve (the tentorium of the optic nerve) which goes from the sphenoid limbus to the anterior clinoid process. In the optic canal, the nerve is attached to the walls through this sheath, which explains why it can be damaged when fractures spread to the canal or when the sinus is infected. All these extensions further strengthen the attachment of the dura mater at the base of the skull.

In the cranial suture regions, fine bundles of vascular and nervous elements in areolar connective tissue emanate from the dura mater and pass via sinuses across the cranium to supply the scalp.

Inner surface

The inner surface of the dura mater sends out extensions which separate the various parts of the encephalon and keep them all in the correct position inside the head.

There are five of these compartments:

- the tentorium cerebelli
- the falx cerebri
- the falx cerebelli
- the diaphragm of sella turcica
- the tentorium of the olfactory bulb

▶ TENTORIUM CEREBELLI

The tentorium cerebelli is a horizontal septum between the superior side of the cerebellum, which it invests, and the lower side of the occipital lobes, which lie over it.

It has two surfaces and two edges. The upper surface is higher in the middle than at the sides due to its insertion at the median line of the falx cerebri. On either side lie the occipital lobes. The lower surface is in the shape of a vault; it lies on the cerebellum and the falx cerebelli is inserted into its median part.

The anterior edge or lesser circumference is markedly concave at the front; it forms the tentorial notch (which is traversed by the brain stem) together with the anterior edge of the basilar pontine sulcus. The anterior edge of each end of the tentorium cerebelli passes over the petrous part of the temporal bone, where it crosses the greater circumference outside the posterior clinoid process and goes on to attach at the top of the lateral edge of the anterior clinoid process.

The ends of the two edges of the tentorium cerebelli form a triangle, the third side of which is represented by a anteroposterior line joining the two clinoid processes. This triangle is filled by a lamina of dura mater in which are buried the oculomotor and trochlear nerves. Extensions emanate from each of the three sides and descend towards the base of the skull where they are solidly attached. They extend from the anterior surface of the petrous part of the temporal bone as far as the superior orbital fissure and the base of the sella turcica. These extensions constitute the medial, lateral, and posterior walls of the cavernous sinus.

The posterior edge (or greater circumference) is concave posteriorly and inserts into the internal occipital protruberance, into the two lips of the sulcus of the lateral sinus, into the upper edge of the petrous part of the temporal bone, and finally into the posterior clinoid process. All along this edge are the lateral sinuses behind and the superior petrosal sinuses on the sides.

Near the top of the petrous part of the temporal bone there is an opening in the posterior edge of the tentorium cerebelli through which passes the trigeminal nerve. This opening gives access to the trigeminal cave, which contains the trigeminal ganglion.

▶ FALX CEREBRI

The falx cerebri is a vertical septum located in the longitudinal cerebral fissure which separates the two hemispheres of the brain.

We will consider its two surfaces, its two edges, its base, and its top. The surfaces cover the internal surfaces of the cerebral hemispheres. The posterior aspect of the base is inclined inferoposteriorly, continuous on the median line with the tentorium cerebelli, which it keeps stretched. The straight sinus runs all the way along the line of intersection between the falx and the tentorium. The anterior aspect of the falx inserts into the crista galli of the ethmoid bone. It sends out an extension into the foramen caecum of the frontal bone.

The upper edge is markedly convex; it occupies the median line from the internal occipital protruberance to the foramen caecum. The superior sagittal sinus is found along this edge. The lower edge is convex and thin. It is apposed to the upper surface of the corpus callosum, but only its posterior part is in direct contact with it. The inferior sagittal sinus is found inside this lower edge.

▶ FALX CEREBELLI

The falx cerebelli is a median, vertically disposed lamina which separates the two hemispheres of the brain:

- Its lateral surfaces are apposed to the cerebellar hemispheres.
- The base, oriented towards the top, joins the median part of the tentorium cerebelli.
- The top, oriented towards the bottom and the front, branches at the level of the foramen magnum with both branches traveling around this opening and continuing on to the jugular foramen. Each contains the lower part of the corresponding posterior occipital sinus.
- The convex posterior edges are inserted into the internal occipital crest and contain the posterior occipital sinuses.
- The free, concave edge of the anterior edge is connected to the vermis cerebelli.

▶ DIAPHRAGMA SELLA

The diaphragma sella is a tensile horizontal septum which is inserted:

- at the upper edge of the posterior aspect of the body of the sphenoid
- to the posterior lip of the prechiasmatic sulcus, and to the four clinoid processes at the front

It joins the wall of the cavernous sinus all along the line at which the superior and medial walls of the sinus meet.

It is composed of two layers:

- a superficial layer, which is the actual diaphragm of sella turcica
- a deep layer, which lines the sella turcica and is continuous with the diaphragm at the prechiasmatic sulcus

The diaphragma sella invests the pituitary gland and is pierced in order to allow passage of the infundibulum hypothalami. It contains the cavernous sinuses.

▶ TENTORIUM OF THE OLFACTORY BULB

This is the name given to a small, crescent-shaped fold of the dura mater which is stretched out on either side of the median line over the anterior end of the olfactory bulb between the crista galli and the anterior edge of the orbital tuberosities of the frontal bone. This structure is often absent.

Innervation

The dura mater of the brain and the scalp are innervated by the trigeminal nerve, the cavernous nervous plexus, and autonomic nerves. Different meningeal rami can be distinguished:

- anterior rami by ethmoidal fibers from the nasal branch of the ophthalmic. One of these meningeal rami, the auricular branch of the vagus nerve, branches off from the ophthalmic nerve and distributes in the tentorium cerebelli. The meningeal ramus of the mandibular nerve passes through the foramen rotundum, and that of the maxillary nerve through the foramen ovale.
- posterior rami via branches of the vagus and the greater hypoglossal nerves, distributing in the dura mater of the posterior fossa, as well as meningeal branches of C1 to C3, which pass through the foramen magnum

Spinal Dura Mater

The spinal dura mater is a fibrous sheath which contains the spinal cord and the spinal roots (Fig. 2-41). It extends from the foramen magnum down to the second sacral vertebra. It fits inside of the vertebral canal. Superiorly it is solidly attached at the third cervical vertebra and around the foramen magnum, where it is continuous with the dura mater of the brain. The vertebral arteries cross it at the atlanto-occipital junction.

Fig. 2-41 Spinal Meninges

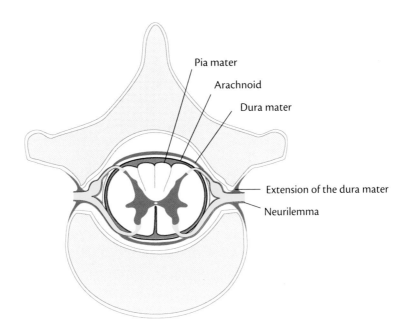

Pia mater

Arachnoid

Dura mater

Extension of the dura mater

Neurilemma

Inferiorly it continues beyond the lower end of the cord to invest all the elements of the cauda equina and the filum terminale. It terminates as a pouch at the second sacral vertebra but continues with the dural part of the filum terminale as far as the coccyx, which is also known as the coccygeal ligament. This ligament is attached to the posterior vertebral ligament by a closed or fenestrated median septum.

The external surface is separated from the walls by the epidural space, which contains veins and semi-fluid lipid material that is especially abundant at the back. The rate of entry and exit of this lipid material depends on the intrathoracic and intra-abdominal pressure.

Posteriorly it is completely free. Anteriorly the epidural space is very narrow and the dura mater is joined to the posterior vertebral ligament by fibrous extensions, which are particularly dense in the cervical and lumbar regions.

Recent dissections have demonstrated the existence of a fibrous, anteroposterior bridge which attaches the dura mater to the atlanto-occipital membrane at the occipital level (Hack, et. al, 1995). Thus, it is continuous with the rectus capitis posterior muscle.

Spinal nerves and roots cross the dura mater, bringing with them extensions of the fascia as far as the intervertebral foramen where, after they have sent out some tracts to the periosteum of the intervertebral foramen, they gradually become continuous with the membrane investing the nerve (Fig. 2-42).

Fig. 2-42   Extensions of spinal meninges

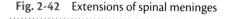

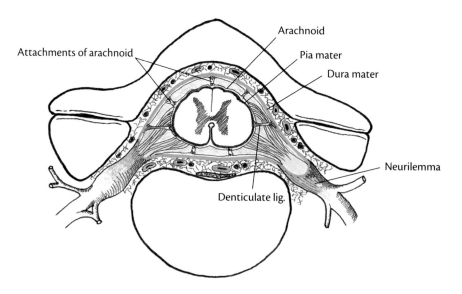

Research has shown that lumbar dural ligaments exist which extend from the dural tube to the common posterior vertebral ligament and from the sulcus of the nerve root to the internal part of the stalk inside the neural canal (Yaszemki and White, 1994). There are also other connections between the dura mater and the nerve roots, above and beyond those listed here. In addition, dural veins are found in these tissues.

The connection between nerve and vertebral ligament arises in the dural sheath of the root at the level of the disk and terminates in the lateral extension of the vertebral ligament. The thickness of this ligament varies at different levels and also between different individuals.

The inner surface covers the parietal layer of the arachnoid membrane. It is joined to the pia mater via a connective tissue tract:

- in the anteroposterior direction, where it is composed of simple filaments
- transversely, where it corresponds to a true membrane which occupies the entire depth of the spinal cord—the denticulate ligament

The purpose of all these extensions is to immobilize and locate the spinal cord at the center of the tube created by the fibrous dura mater, and to enhance its protection.

The dura mater of the spinal cord is innervated by the meningeal branch of spinal nerves.

PIA MATER

The pia mater is the innermost of the three meningeal membranes. It is a cellulovascular structure. The pia mater forms a special sheath called the neurilemma, which invests all the nerves emanating from the cranium and the spinal cord and follows them until their termination.

Cerbral Pia Mater

The pia mater of the brain is thinner, more amply supplied with blood, and less strongly attached to other structures than its spinal cord portion.

The pia mater covers the external surface of the encephalon and insinuates itself into all its depths and sulci. It is more strongly attached at the protruberance and peduncles than at the cerebellum or cerebrum. At the same time, it is less vascular and stronger.

The inner surface is in direct contact with the nervous tissue and is loosely attached to it via connecting filaments and, more importantly, by the myriad tiny vessels which cross in both directions between the two tissues.

The external surface is connected to the sub-arachnoid space through which circulates the cerebrospinal fluid. At the level of the great transverse cerebral fissure (Bichat's fissure), the pia mater of the brain insinuates itself into the interior brain to form the telae choroideae ventriculi and the choroid plexi.

Spinal Pia Mater

This is continuous with the pia mater of the brain and extends at the bottom around the filum terminale as the coccygeal ligament, which inserts at the base of the coccyx. This ligament is small but very strong and is important in immobilizing the lowermost end of the spinal cord.

The inner surface is attached to all parts of the underlying nervous tissue by means of numerous connective tissue septa which penetrate into the white matter. It also sends out extensions into the posterior and anterior median sulci. The external surface is bathed in cerebrospinal fluid. It is connected to the dura mater via both anteroposterior and lateral extensions.

There are are tiny emanations of connective tissue, particularly small at the front but denser and stronger at the back, known as anteroposterior extensions. They form a septum on the median line which is particularly complete in the thoracolumbar region.

The deticulate ligaments of the spinal cord are lateral extensions that extend transversely from the pia mater to the dura mater, starting at the lateral masses of the atlas bone and as far as the first lumbar vertebra. They are located between the anterior and posterior roots of the spinal nerves. The lateral edge is scalloped or dentellate, with the projections attaching to the dura mater between the openings for the two neighboring spinal nerves. Between each pair of projections, the lateral edge of the ligament is free and allows the passage of the roots of the same spinal nerve. The most cephalic of the dentate ligaments is attached to the vertebral artery and the hypoglossal nerve near the foramen magnum.

ARACHNOID MEMBRANE

The arachnoid membrane is a thin connective tissue membrane found between the pia mater and the dura mater. It is tightly associated with the latter at all points. It defines two spaces, namely, the subdural and the subarachnoid spaces.

The more or less virtual subdural space is crossed by numerous arteries, veins, and nerve fibers which are entering or leaving the central nervous system. In its spinal portion, it is also crossed by various trabeculae of connective tissue and the denticulate ligaments which join the pia mater to the dura mater.

The arachnoid membrane first appears in the embryo between days twelve and thirteen. At thirty weeks, it is still thin and often incomplete, but it is stronger by week thirty-eight. It continues to thicken and elaborate more connections throughout fetal development and for three years after birth. The dentate ligament of the spinal cord first appears around day forty-one.

Cerebral Arachnoid Membrane

The visceral layer of the arachnoid membrane is apposed to the dura mater and does not follow the pia mater in its invaginations into the sulci and fissures of the brain, but rather passes flat over them. Here, the sub-arachnoid spaces are enlarged, forming cavities where varying volumes of cerebrospinal fluid can accumulate (Fig. 2-43).

These cavities are called cisterns. Among the most important are the:

- chiasmatic cistern (also known as the cistern of the lamina terminalis), in front of the optic chiasm
- pontine cistern, which is lower down on the ventral surface of the pons
- supracallosal cistern, which is superior to the corpus callosum
- cerebellomedullary cistern (also known as the cisterna magna), between the medulla oblongata and the cerebellum
- interpenducular cistern, between the two cerbral peduncles
- cistern of the great cerebral vein (also known as the superior cistern), in the middle portion of the transverse cerebral fissure

Fig. 2-43   Cerbral cisterns

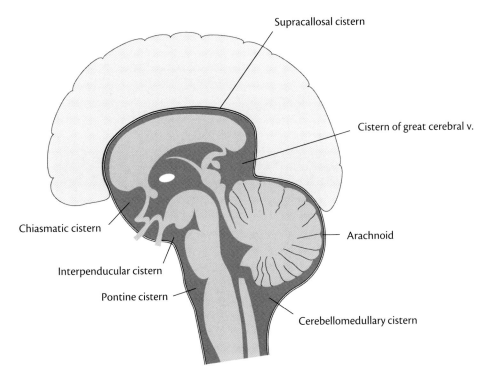

The arachnoid membrane of the brain contains arachnoid granulations (also known as pacchionian bodies), which are small elevations concentrated around the sinuses and representing the structures through which the cerebrospinal fluid is reabsorbed. These granulations grow from the inside towards the outside, obeying a force which pushes them out to come into contact with the inner wall of the cranium. There they can create depressions on the inner surface of the skull called granular foveolae. These can be deep, especially in the elderly, and can even, in a very small number of extreme cases, pierce the top of the skull and project out just below the integument.

Spinal Arachnoid Membrane

This is continuous with the arachnoid membrane of the brain at the foramen magnum and extends to the cauda equina, tightly associated with the dura mater at all points. It lines all the vessels, nerves, and dentate ligaments, and travels with the nerve roots as far as the intervertebral foramen, where it folds back on itself. Parts of the inner surface of the arachnoid membrane are doubled up by a supplementary membrane, the leptomeninx (Nicholas and Weller, 1988; Parkinson, 1991).

The leptomeninx is found at the level of the spinal cord but not in the cerebrum (Fig. 2-44). It is most obvious in the thoracic region. The sub-arachnoid space is separated from the perivascular spaces (Virchow-Robin spaces) by a layer of pia mater in the spinal column, but not in the brain.

Fig. 2-44 Cross-section through the Spinal Cord and its Meninges

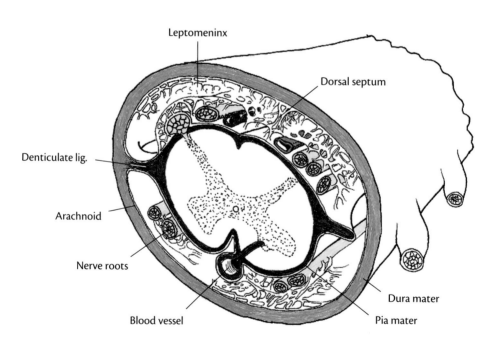

The leptomeninx lines the innermost surface of the median arachnoid membrane and folds back on itself at the median line to form posterior septa, which loosely link the arachnoid membrane and the pia mater. It should be noted that a lateral septum is found at the thoracic level.

This leptomeninx also lines the pia mater and the dentate ligaments. The collagen fibers in the dentate ligaments are thicker on the dura mater side than they are on the pia mater side. The leptomeninx is a fenestrated structure and contains trabeculae, which are attached to the nerves and vessels of the pia mater as well as to the pia mater itself. The pia mater is joined to the spinal cord by groups of collagen fibers which are denser at the thoracic level, but these attachments are not fenestrated.

A fenestrated but less obvious leptomeninx structure is also found at the ventral level, surrounding the anterior spinal artery. No septa have ever been observed in this region.

The leptomeninx and the ligaments are more pronounced in humans, probably because of our ability to take an erect position. The reason for the fenestrated configuration around vessels is almost certainly related to the damping of pressure waves generated when changing posture. The fenestration would also be useful in maintaining the stability of the nerves, vessels, and spinal cord in the sub-arachnoid space.

The leptomeninx defines a space between itself and the pia mater in which cerebrospinal fluid circulates. At the spinal cord level, the fluid is reabsorbed via the perivenous sheaths and the paravertebral lymph nodes.

The arachnoid membrane and the pia mater of the brain are innervated by the nervous plexuses which are associated with the vessels.

Table 2-12 Connections of the Meninges

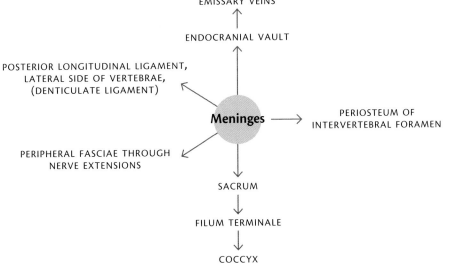

Fig. 2-45   Overall Arrangement of the Fasciae with Points of Continuity

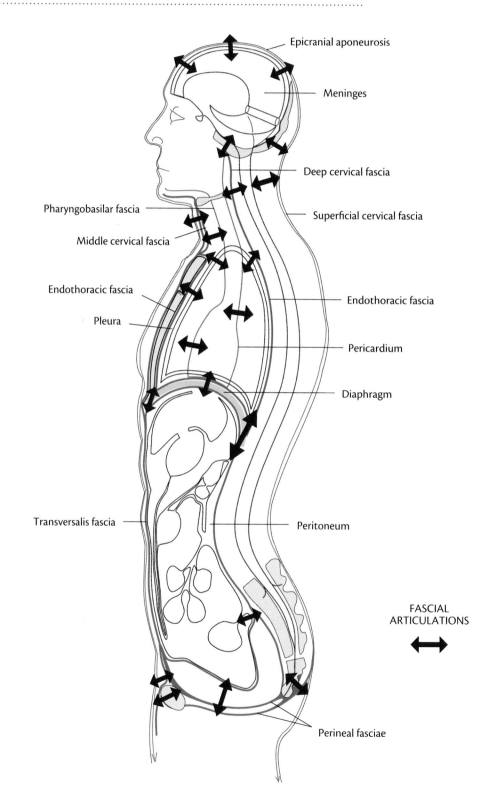

3

Connective Tissue Anatomy at the Microscopic Level

"A tissue can be defined as the first level of multicellular organization: it corresponds to a group of differentiated cells which together form a unit that is a territorial, functional and physiological entity."

—J. Racadot, *Précis D'Histologie Humaine*

IN THIS CHAPTER we will briefly go over the microscopic anatomy of the connective tissue. This background will help in understanding some of the subtleties of fascial techniques and place them in a global perspective. As noted in Coujard et. al., Bernandin and Kaiyos proposed a biochemical definition of connective tissue based on the presence of four specific types of macromolecules: collagen, elastin, proteoglycans, and structural glycoproteins. In connective tissue, interactions among stationary cels, motile cells, and a matrix create a relatively loosely structured network. The bound cells are named according to the type of tissue in which they are found, that is, connective cells, cartilage cells, bone cells, etc. (Fig. 3-1). The matrix or interstitial substance is made up of a ground substance and various types of fibers.

Distinction is made among the following types of tissues:

- Connective tissues
  - mesenchyme
  - reticular tissue
  - interstitial tissue
  - fibrous tissue
  - adipose tissue
- Cartilaginous tissues
  - hyaline cartilage
  - elastic cartilage
  - fibrocartilage
  - bone

Fig. 3-1 Origins of Connective Tissues

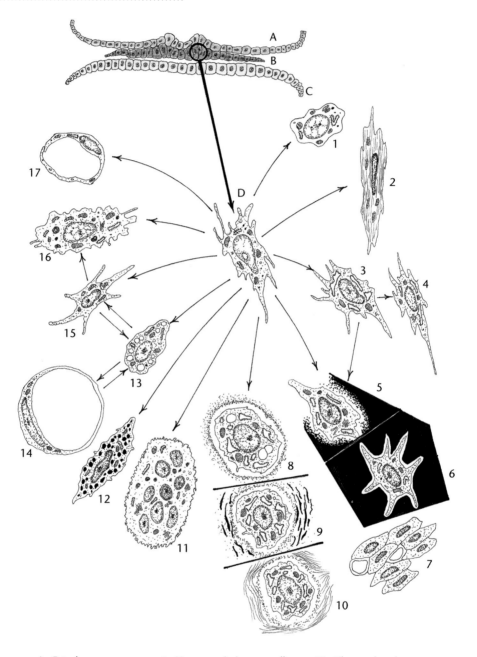

A	Ectoderm	1	Hematopoietic stem cells	10	Fibrous chondrocyte
B	Mesoderm	2	Smooth m. cells	11	Chondroclasts
C	Endoderm	3	Fibroblasts	12	Mast cells
D	Mesenchymal cell	4	Fibrocytes	13	Lipoblasts
		5	Osteoblasts	14	Adipocytes
		6	Osteocytes	15	Reticular cells
		7	Odontoblasts	16	Macrophages
		8	Hyaline chondrocyte	17	Endothelial cells
		9	Elastic chondrocyte		

Connective Tissues

As stated above, conventionally there are distinctions made among the different types of connective tissue. In reality there is no clear demarcation line between one type and another, and they can all be considered different densities of the same tissue. The key physical and mechanical properties of connective tissue are:

- elasticity
- viscosity
- plasticity
- strength

Connective tissue is made up of various types of cells supported in an interstitial matrix.

CONNECTIVE TISSUE CELLS

Bound cells

- fibrocytes (a mature form of fibroblast)
- mesenchymal cells
- reticular cells
- pigment cells
- adipocytes

Unbound cells

- macrophages
- mast cells (the most abundant)
- lymphocytes
- plasma cells
- granulocytes

Interstitial matrix

This matrix mainly consists of a network of different fibers.

Reticular fibers

Similar in structure to collagen fibers, reticular fibers form a network around the blood capillaries and are found in the basal substance in the urinary ducts.

Collagen fibers

Made up of groups of fibrils held together by an amorphous cement. They are relatively inextensible and are always found in the tissues in the form of bundles of fibers. They are especially abundant in the tendons, the tympanic membrane, and certain fasciae.

Elastic fibers

Found in many connective tissues, for example, in the coronary arteries and certain ligaments, like the ligamenta flava.

Ground substance

This is largely secreted *in situ* by connective tissue cells and plays an important role in homeostasis, notably in the metabolic exchange processes which occur between cells and the blood.

Various types of connective tissue

Mesenchyma

This is the embryonic connective tissue.

Reticular tissue

Distinction is made between:

- lymphoid tissue (lymph nodes)
- myeloid tissue (bone marrow)

Interstitial tissue

Interstitial tissue, or stroma, is rather loosely structured. Its function is to pack the spaces and provide a lubricating layer between other structures (e.g., muscles and internal organs).

The stroma plays an important role in many metabolic processes, notably in tissue regeneration. It contains:

- collagen fibers
- elastic fibers
- reticular fibers
- ground substance
- cells

Fibrous tissue

Fibrous or dense connective tissue contains a particularly high proportion of collagen fibers, with a lower density of cells and less ground substance than in stroma. This is the form of connective tissue found in tendons as well as the plantar and volar fasciae.

Adipose tissue

Distinction is usually made between two different types:

- white adipose tissue,
- brown adipose tissue

The latter type is highly represented in new-borns. In adult humans, it is only found in certain specific parts of the body (e.g., the adipose capsule of the kidney).

Adipose tissue is composed of adipocytes suspended in an interstitial matrix. Distinction is usually made between:

- fat storage tissue, the quantity of which depends on nutritional status, mostly found in subcutaneous cushions where it is ready for consumption when energy is needed
- structural adipose tissue, the quantity of which is independent of nutritional status, which is found in such places as the:
  — joints
  — bone marrow
  — adipose tissue of the cheek

CARTILAGINOUS TISSUE

Cartilaginous tissue is made up of cells in a highly hydrated (70% water) interstitial substance which contains hardly any vessels or nerves. It is the nature of the interstitial substance which defines the different types of cartilaginous tissue, with distinction usually made among:

- hyaline cartilage
- elastic cartilage
- fibrocartilage

Hyaline cartilage

This form consists of an interstitial substance containing small collagen fibrils and isolated networks of elastic fibers. Most of the body's cartilaginous tissues are invested by a continuous extension called the perichondrium. This type of cartilage is found in the joints, the costal articulations, the airways, connecting cartilage, and the skeletal frame.

Elastic cartilage

The interstitial substance of elastic cartilage contains a higher proportion of elastic fibers and fewer collagen fibrils than hyaline cartilage. This is found in such tissues as the pinna of the ear and the epiglottis.

Fibrocartilage

Fibrocartilage contains few cells but is rich in collagen fibers. It is notably found in the intervertebral disks and the ligaments associated with the pubic symphysis.

The intervertebral disks are kept in place by hyaline cartilage which is strongly attached to the bodies of the vertebrae. The disk extends from the inner face of the vertebral body and adheres to thin layers of hyaline cartilage. When a disk ruptures through the vertebral end plate, it forms structures known as Schmorl's nodes.

The posterior longitudinal ligament is strongly attached to the disk. At this point, we find a fascial continuity between cartilaginous, fibrous, and bony tissue.

BONY TISSUE

Bony tissue is composed of:

- bone cells or osteocytes
- ground substance
- collagen fibrils
- a cement substance
- various salts

All bony tissue is based on just two fundamental components, namely, ground substance and collagen fibrils. Therefore, bony tissue can be thought of as a fascia which has undergone thorough consolidation. The fibrils represent one of the organic constituents of bone (as opposed to the salts, which are the mineral constituents).

The strength of bone partially depends on its organic components, and when these are deficient, it loses elasticity and tends to break easily. Therefore, bone, like all the other types of fascia, is characterized by three key properties—elasticity, plasticity, and strength.

Different types of bony tissue

Distinction is made between two different types of bony tissue on the basis of how the fibrils are organized:

- reticular bony tissue
- lamellar or haversian bony tissue

Reticular bony tissue

Reticular bony tissue is formed when connective tissue is converted into bone. It is most abundant during development, but persists into adulthood around the cranial sutures.

Lamellar bony tissue

Lamellar bony tissue accounts for all the other bones in the body. It is clearly stratified with lamellae of ground substance alternating with layers of osteocytes. These layers are organized concentrically around a haversian canal to form the basic unit of compact bone, the osteon (Fig. 3-2). Neighboring osteons are separated by interstitial lamellae. The longitudinal haversian canals are interconnected by the more or less obliquely inclined Volkmann's canals.

The way in which the osteons are constructed and organized depends on the load borne by the specific bone. In this manner the tissue is characterized by the same kind of variability and adaptation as the fasciae.

The formation of bone is mediated by osteoblasts, specialized mesenchymal cells (the cells from which all tissues are derived). The osteoblasts secrete osteoid, a special kind of interstitial substance composed of a soft ground substance and collagen fibers.

Fig. 3-2   Two Osteocytes and Part of an Osteon

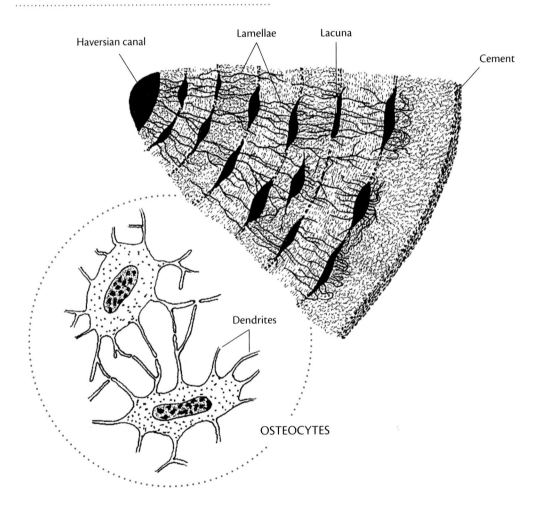

Various types of ossification

Distinction is usually made between two different modes of ossification:

- endoconnective ossification; also known as direct or fibrous ossification
- cartilaginous ossification; also known as indirect ossification, as it involves the replacement of pre-existing cartilage

Endoconnective ossification

This refers to the formation of bone from connective tissue. The nature of the bone, initially fibrous, gradually changes to a lamellar structure. This type of ossification is found in:

- the bones of the calvaria
- the facial bones
- the clavicle

Cartilaginous ossification

Cartilaginous ossification describes the process in which pre-existing cartilaginous structures are replaced with bony tissue. This process involves cells called chondroclasts, which absorb the cartilage and thus allow its replacement with bony tissue produced by osteoblasts.

Distinction is usually made between two different forms of cartilaginous ossification:

- endochondral ossification, which occurs within the cartilage around the epiphyses
- perichondral ossification, which progresses from the perichondrium and only occurs in the diaphyses

Periosteum

The periosteum is a fibrous, elastic membrane which covers the entire bone apart from its cartilaginous portions. It is continuous with both the fascial sheets and the tendons which attach the muscles to the bones (further evidence of the uninterrupted continuity of the fascial system).

The strength of attachment of the periosteum to the bone varies enormously:

- It is very tightly attached to short bones.
- It is less strongly attached to long bones, although in these bones the association tends to be tighter at the epiphysis than along the diaphysis.

These characteristics of the periosteum are due to the presence of:

- tendons and fasciae, which have the effect of fixing the periosteum to the bone mass
- nerves and vessels extending from the periosteum into the bone, which similarly hold the two tissues together
- Sharpey's fibers, which are connecting fibers that emanate from the periosteum and are embedded in the bone (another example of fascial continuity: from the periosteum to the bone where all fasciae terminate)

Inner periosteal surface

Vessels and nerves project from the inner surface of the periosteum into the bone.

Also on this surface is a layer of endosteum, which is involved in the radial growth of bones.

Outer periosteal surface

It is the outer surface of the periosteum which is in contact with the muscles, tendons, and fasciae. In certain places, this tissue is very close to the skin with just a simple fascia or thin, sparse cellular layer separating the two (e.g., at the tibia and the zygomatic bone).

Structure

Distinction is usually made between two different layers in this fibrous tissue:

- an external layer of connective tissue, which is rich in elastic fibers
- a deep layer based on similar but finer components

The deep layer is the thinner of the two and its network of elastic fibers is woven more tightly. Connective and elastic fibers (sometimes known as archiform Ranvier fibers) project from this inner surface and are embedded in the bone.

One of the functions located in the deep layer is the generation of osteoblasts. These generally disappear once growth is finished but they can return at any time to regenerate bony tissue following damage.

The periosteum is highly vascular and provides all the nutritional elements which are needed by bone. If the periosteum is destroyed, the bone becomes necrotic. The periosteum is innervated by a very dense network of nerve fibers, which accounts for its exquisite sensitivity. Some of these fibers pass over into the bony tissue in association with blood vessels. The periosteum also contains a dense network of lymphatics.

Organization of bony tissue

Bony tissue consists of cells (osteoblasts, osteocytes, and osteoclasts) in a matrix.

Matrix

The matrix consists of an organic ground substance containing mineralized collagen fibers and a variety of mineral salts.

▶ ORGANIC MATRIX

This consists of:

- a very dense network of collagen fibers. Tubular fibrils which are present within bony tissue have been shown to be extensions of fibrils in the tendons and fasciae which are inserted into the bone—these are called Sharpey's fibers.
- a ground substance, which is relatively sparse and contains a variety of different mucopolysaccharides, glycoproteins, and structural proteins as well as water and electrolytes

▶ MINERAL SALTS

It is its mineral content which makes bony tissue hard, especially crystalline hydroxyapatite, a salt containing calcium and phosphate.

Deposition and reabsorption of bony tissue

Throughout life, bony tissue is subject to continuous turnover, a process which involves both catabolism and anabolism.

▶ DEPOSITION

A bony tissue precursor substance, a mixture of glycoproteins, mucopolysaccharides, and tropocollagen, is synthesized and secreted by osteoblasts. This precursor substance then becomes mineralized by the deposition of calcium phosphate, which subsequently crystallizes in the form of hydroxyapatite.

▶ REABSORPTION

Two processes are involved in the reabsorption of bony tissue:

- osteoclast-mediated reabsorption, which is stimulated by the local presence of parathyroid hormone. Osteoclasts secrete a variety of effector molecules: H+ ions which attack the mineral material; acid hydrolase enzymes which break down glycoproteins and mucopolysaccharides, and collagenase enzymes which break down collagen.
- periosteocytic reabsorption: certain osteoclasts are particularly lytically active and induce demineralization and lysis of surrounding bony tissue

Related Tissues

To conclude this section, we will briefly review certain features of other tissues that are very closely associated with the connective tissues. The connective tissues provide these other tissues with both physical and material support.

MUSCLE

Muscle tissue cannot be considered independently of the fascial system which completely invests all the muscles of the body and provides both reinforcment and insertion points. Moreover, like all fasciae, those which invest muscles act as a conduit for the nerves and vessels without which the muscles could not function.

A muscle is constructed of a series of different levels of fibers (Fig. 3-3). Each level is invested by a specific type of connective tissue. The muscle as a whole is surrounded with an element of the fascial system called the epimysium. The epimysium divides to form the septa of the perimysial network which invest the primary fascicles. The perimysium further divides to form the connective tissue covering which defines each separate muscle fiber, the endomysium. Finally, each muscle fiber is composed of a group of myofibrils. The myofibril corresponds to the most basic unit of muscle tissue and is covered by a delicate membrane called the sarcolemma.

Fig. 3-3   Skeletal Muscle Structure

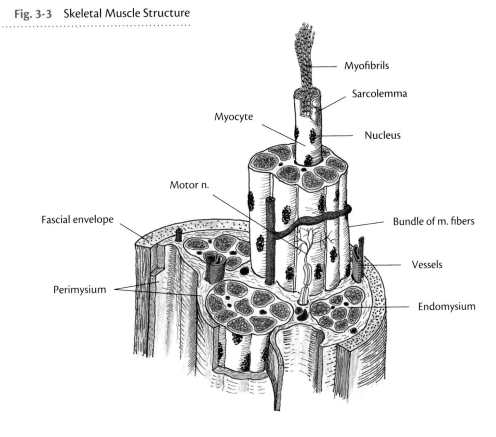

Extensions continuous with the muscle tissue project from the ends of muscles to form the tendons where fasciae or membranes converge to form a thick cord which is both extremely strong and elastic.

Tendons are formed of two different types of connective tissue:

- fibrous tissue
- loose cellular tissue

The basic unit of the tendon is a primary bundle of fibers grouped together inside a sheath. These primary bundles group with one another to form secondary bundles, which define another level of fiber. The secondary bundles, in turn, group together to form a tertiary structure, the tendon itself, which is invested with a third level of membrane.

In certain tendinous bodies, some of the softer connective tissue has been replaced by true bony tissue—these are the so-called sesamoid bones, the most remarkable of which is the patella.

Two different types of muscle tissue are recognized:

- smooth muscle
- striated muscle

Smooth muscle tissue

These have:

- a central nucleus
- myofilament-containing cytoplasm
- a plasma membrane covered in a basement membrane into which are inserted bundles of collagen fibers

Striated muscle tissue

Each of these cells contains several hundred nuclei located against the plasma membrane, with the whole syncytium covered in a basement membrane.

Muscle fibers are assembled in bundles together with interstitial, highly vascular connective tissue. Muscles are attached to skeletal elements via aponeuroses and tendons based on collagen fibers emanating from the end of each myocyte.

NERVES

Nerves are composed of conducting nerve cells together with a mesenchymal system for their support and protection.

Central nervous system

The tissue which invests and provides support for the central nervous system is called the neuroglia. This tissue is made up of modified ectodermal elements and it fulfills the conventional functions of connective tissue, that is, it provides physical support, a medium for the exchange of materials, and, when pathological processes are active, mediates reabsorption and repair.

Three different types of cells are involved in this system:

Astrocytes

Protoplasmic astrocytes are more abundant in the gray matter while fibrillary astrocytes predominate in the white matter and have long, thin cytoplasmic processes. After the destruction of central nervous tissue, they form glial scar tissue.

The astrocytes fulfill a supporting role and are found around the periphery of the brain where they form the glial membrane. They send processes out to nearby blood vessels. The walls of these vessels, together with the basement membrane, separate the ectodermal cerebral tissue from the mesodermal capillary tissue, that is, these structures constitute the blood-brain barrier which blocks the passage from the blood of materials which are not wanted in the brain. Astrocytes are relatively immobile.

Oligodendroglia

Oligodendrocytes associate with nerve cells in the gray matter; in white matter they are found in rows between the nerve fibers and are believed to be involved in myelin production. Their cell bodies are constantly pulsating—alternately contracting and dilating—with a regular rhythm.

Microglia

When nervous tissue is damaged, these cells phagocytose any debris, changing shape when they do so. They are highly motile and rapidly move around between the cytoplasmic processes of the astrocytes, constantly changing shape.

The neuroglia invests and protects the neurons which correspond to the basic unit of the central nervous system. A typical neuron consists of a cell body (the cell's active metabolic center), a number of relatively short, radiating processes (the dendrites), and one principal process (the axon) which conducts the nervous signal and which may or may not be surrounded by a myelinated Schwann cell sheath. The central part of a nerve cell contains the semi-fluid cytoplasm, which is continuously flowing away from the cell body.

Peripheral nervous system

The basic unit of the peripheral nervous system is the nerve fiber. At the center of a nerve fiber is the axon of a nerve cell, the body of which is implanted in either the spinal cord or one of the craniospinal ganglia. This axon is surrounded by a cellular sheath from which it may or may not be separated by a layer of myelin. This, in turn, is enclosed in a connective tissue sheath (the endoneurium) that is made up of longitudinally disposed collagen fibrils which, together with the basement membrane, form the endoneural membrane or neurilemma.

Individual nerve cells are bundled together to form fascicles or funiculi, which represent the functional anatomical unit of the nerve. Within the fascicle, the cells are supported in a special areolar connective tissue structure called the endoneurium. The fascicles are invested by the perineurium, which is mainly composed of longitudinally disposed fibers, although the presence of some circular elastic fibers in this layer helps make peripheral nerves resistant to physical stress. In the limbs, the perineurium is reinforced around the joints.

The entire nerve (consisting of one or more fascicles) is invested by the epineurium, a special areolar connective tissue structure which also contains fatty tissue, blood vessels, and lymphatics (Fig. 3-4). Each nerve makes its way to its ultimate destination in association with a fascial support structure which protects it and keeps it supplied with blood over its entire length.

Therefore, each nerve consists of a connective tissue sheath (the epineurium) enclosing bundles (fascicles) of nerve fibers, each bundle in turn surrounded by its own connective tissue sheath called the perineurium. Each individual fiber in a bundle has its own distinct type of connective tissue sheath called the endoneurium. The perineurium acts as a barrier to diffusion and separates the epineurium (which has a protective role) from the endoneurium.

Fig. 3-4   Cross-section through a Nerve and Associated Fascial Elements

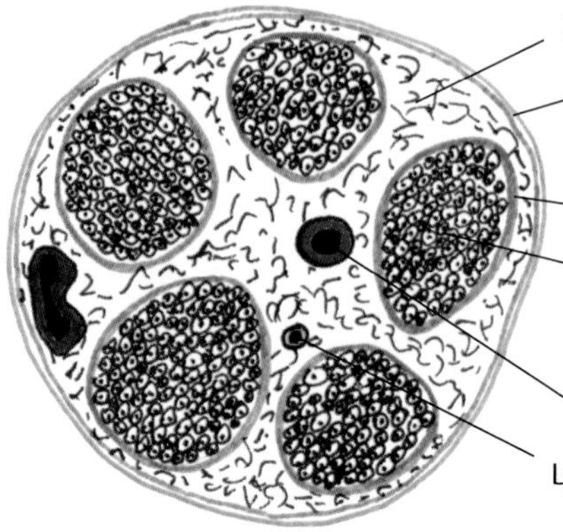

Epineurium
Neurilemma
Perineurium
Endoneurium
Arterial capillary
Lymphatic vessel

EPITHELIAL LINING

The tissues of the epithelial lining are composed of tightly-packed cells which form sheets covering the entire outer surface of the body and lining all the internal cavities of the body.

System of intercellular junctions

Neighboring cells are joined to one another by interdigitations of their plasma membranes but, more importantly, via special cell-cell junction structures which hold the epithelial sheets together with remarkable efficiency. There are three different types of epithelial junction:

Tight or occluding junctions

The two adjacent plasma membranes are very tightly joined via linear arrays of transmembrane proteins on each cell which lock into one another, analogous to how a zipper works.

Adherent junctions

Adherent junctions are based on the presence of adhesive-like material between adjacent cells.

Gap junctions

Adjacent cells are joined through pores which are created by transmembrane proteins which come together to form a channel; these pores allow the direct transfer of material between the cells.

Relationships between epithelial and connective tissue

The apical surface of any internal epithelium is in direct contact with the lumen of the cavity it is lining, whereas its basal surface rests on some form of connective tissue with a sheet of amorphous extracellular material in between, called the basement membrane (Fig. 3-5). It functions as a supporting structure with variations in tension, and as a barrier. In this way it can influence filtration, diffusion, and exchange processes.

Basement membranes are comprised of two distinct layers:

- an upper layer, the basal lamina, which is composed of glycoproteins and type IV collagen
- a deeper layer, the reticular lamina, which is composed of reticular fibers

Fig. 3-5 Links Between Fasciae and Capillaries

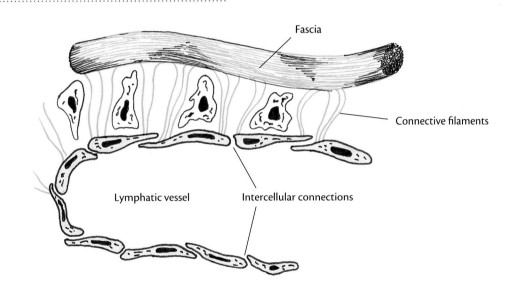

Fascia

Connective filaments

Lymphatic vessel   Intercellular connections

Cell differentiation and functional specialization

Different epithelia have different functions and correspondingly consist of different cell types to mediate these diverse functions. Epithelial cells have a short lifetime and epithelia are regenerated from undifferentiated cells which form the layer in contact with the basement membrane. The different cell types include:

- the keratinized cells of the epidermis, which play an important protective role
- the pigment cells of the retina, which produce melanin to protect against UV radiation
- sensory cells and primary sensory neurons, like those found in the inner ear and in the systems involved in the senses of taste and smell
- epithelial cells, which are involved in exchange processes, such as those making up the mesothelial surfaces of the serous membranes and the epithelia of the alveoli of the lungs

- ciliated cells, in the airways and the ducts of the genital system, such as the uterine tubes
- gland cells
- cells which are specialized in absorption processes, such as those in striated membranes which make up the lining of the renal tubules

SKIN

The skin covers the entire external surface of the body and has a total area of about 1.6 square meters. Around the body openings, the skin is continuous with the mucous membranes.

Various layers of the skin

Distinction is usually made between three different layers (Fig. 3-6). Going from the most superficial inwards, these are:

- the epidermis
- the dermis
- the subcutaneous fascia

Fig. 3-6   The Skin
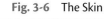

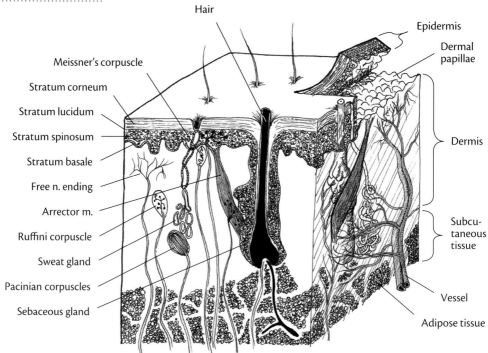

Epidermis

The epidermis is a stratified, keratinized epithelium composed of a variable number of layers. The cells of the epidermis accomplish their migration from the layer adjacent to the basement membrane out to the surface within a period of about thirty days. Going from the deepest layer outwards, the layers of this tissue include:

- the stratum basale: This layer of cells rests on a basement membrane which separates the epidermis from the dermis. Numerous projections extend into the dermis, anchoring the basal layer cells and providing a surface for exchange (especially of nutrients).
- the stratum spinosum: In this layer, the spaces between cells are greater and the cells are full of tonofibrils, which confer stability.
- the stratum lucidum, where eleidin and keratin first appear
- the stratum corneum, where keratinization and desquamation take place

Dermis

Due to its abundance of collagen fibers, the dermis is the part which is responsible for most of the skin's physical strength. Leather is derived from the dermis. The elasticity of the skin is mainly due to the changes in angle between the different planes in the dermis. Networks of elastic fibers insure reintegration of the fibrous layers after they have been deformed. It is the transverse links which allow the return to normal after the skin has been folded over on itself or deformed. As the fibers age, the links weaken and this results in the flaccidity and wrinkling seen in adulthood and old age.

The dermis contains the hair follicles, various types of glands, blood vessels, connective tissue cells, migrating immune system cells, and a variety of nervous system structures. It consists of two layers:

- the stratum papillare
- the stratum reticulare

▶ STRATUM PAPILLARE

The papillary dermis lies immediately below the epidermal basement membrane and is linked to the epidermis through reticular fibers emanating from the bottommost layer of epidermal cells.

▶ STRATUM RETICULARE

The reticular dermis contains a dense network of cross-linked collagen fibers and it is this layer which makes skin tissue resistant to tearing and breakage.

The fibers of the dermis tend to be oriented in a specific direction so that if the skin is perforated, the resultant wound tends to be in the form of an elongated window rather than a symmetrical hole. Surgeons are familiar with and exploit this 'grain', preferring to make their incisions parallel to the fibers rather than across them, because wounds made in this way tend to heal more quickly.

Extreme stress will tear fibers and lead to the appearance of permanent stretch marks.

Subcutaneous tissue

The subcutaneous tissue, or subcutis, is a loosely structured fascia which is continuous with the dermis and provides lubrication between the different layers. It acts as a fat storage tissue in which the stored fat also provides thermal insulation. The status of the subcutaneous adipose tissue reserves is under hormonal control.

The subcutaneous tissue overlies the superficial fascia except where the latter is not present, notably on the face where the subcutaneous tissue is in direct contact with the muscles (which makes grimacing and other facial expression all the easier).

Skin functions

Protective function

The skin protects the body from chemical, physical, and thermal insults, as well as against attack from a wide range of pathogenic agents.

Immune function

The skin is rich in immunocompetent cells and is an important immune organ.

Thermal regulation

The skin helps regulate internal body temperature by modulating blood flow through surface vessels and through the perspiration response.

Regulation of the body's fluid balance

The skin both protects against water loss and also mediates the elimination of small amounts of excess water and electrolytes in perspiration.

Sensory function

By virtue of its many nervous structures, the skin is sensitive to pressure, temperature, and pain. It is also important in communication through its capacity to turn red or white, and its horripilation response. The electrical resistance of the skin changes under the influence of emotional stress. Finally, the skin reflects and acts as an indicator of what is happening in the deeper tissues, especially in terms of the composition of the ground substance.

Hartmut Heine, who participated in the work on the importance of the ground substance with Alfred Pischinger, showed that the ground substance sends out extensions towards the surface in the form of cylinders surrounding nerves and blood vessels. These 'Heine cylinders' modify the structure of the skin and may represent a sensory organ for magnetic and electromagnetic forces. Such a phenomenon may explain how stimulation of the skin could induce long term modification of internal regulatory processes. This cylinder system represents a fascial component which puts the deep fasciae in communication with the surface "in a visible fashion."

Histological Features of Connective Tissue

Connective tissue is a heterogenous mix of various cells and fibers as well as background materials (Fig. 3-7).

CONSTITUENTS OF CONNECTIVE TISSUE

Ground substance

Ground substance is a homogenous medium which can vary in consistency from fluid to semi-fluid (i.e., a gel). It is a colloidal solution of various mucopolysaccharides—including both sulfated species (e.g., chondroitin sulfate and heparin sulfate) and non-sulfated species (e.g., hyaluronic acid), and is rich in proteoglycans and structural glycoproteins.

The binding of variable quantities of water in the tissue space induces changes in the viscosity of ground substance. A viscous ground substance helps prevent the spread of pathogenic agents, and the degree of viscosity also influences the metabolic activity of cells in the vicinity. At body temperature, half of the bound water is in the form of liquid crystals.

The ground substance provides a highly hydrated environment for the fibrous proteins thereby helping them fulfill their various roles in lubrication, shock absorption, and resistance to compressive forces. By virtue of their electrical charge, the components of the ground substance also affect a variety of other factors, both within the connective tissue and outside of it.

Ground substance is key in cellular nutrition because it provides the exchange medium for substances diffusing out of the dense capillary network into the surrounding tissue. The proteoglycans and structural proteins form a molecular sieve through which must pass anything that is exchanged in either direction between the cell and the circulatory system. Species which are either too large or which carry an incompatible electrical charge are filtered out, that is, either excluded or retained. The pore size of this molecular filter depends on the concentration of proteoglycans in that specific connective tissue compartment. The overall negative charge of the proteoglycans insures that the ground substance is both isosmotic and isotonic at all times.

The ground substance of connective tissue can be considered as the laboratory in which all the diverse jobs of the tissue are taken care of.

Collagens

Collagen is the most abundant of all the proteins found in the human body and accounts for 60 to 70% of the overall mass of connective tissue. Tropocollagen is the basic sub-unit from which all forms of collagen are built.

Tropocollagen

Tropocollagen is extremely rich in glycine, which distinguishes it (along with elastin) from other proteins found in the body. One quarter of all the amino acids in tropocollagen are derived from proline.

Collagen synthesis

Most of the body's collagen is synthesized by fibroblasts, although it can also be produced by smooth muscle cells, and endothelial and epithelial cells. Protocollagen is first synthesized on endoplasmic reticulum-bound ribosomes, and then its proline and lysine residues are hydroxylated by the action of two enzymes, tropocollagen-proline-hydroxylase and tropocollagen-lysine-hydroxylase. Next, its hydroxy groups and some of its hydroxylysine groups are glycosylated by conjugation with sugar residues (galactose or glucosylgalactose). Once they have been released from the ribosome, three a-chains of protocollagen are aligned in parallel and then helically coiled together to form the protocollagen sub-unit.

Protocollagen seems to be transported out of the cell via Golgi vesicles and/or vesicles which bud off from the endoplasmic reticulum.

The extracellular process of fibrillogenesis involves cleavage and results in the release of functional tropocollagen. This cleavage reaction can be incomplete, as is known to be the case in the type of collagen found in basement membranes.

Tropocollagen then undergoes polymerization to form fibrils. This process seems to depend on the amount of carbohydrate associated with the tropocollagen molecule, with the rate of fibril formation being inversely proportional to the quantity of sugar (the type of collagen found in basement membranes is particularly rich in carbohydrate and does not form fibrils).

Extracellular maturation to form fibrils and collagen fibers is mainly dependent on the amount of proteoglycan and glycosaminoglycan in the environment.

Collagen is highly resistant to the action of all proteolytic enzymes and is only broken by certain specific collagenase activities.

The rate of collagen turnover varies enormously between different tissues. It is very low in stable tissues, but it can be very high in certain situations (e.g., during wound healing and in the uterus during gestation).

Types of collagen

Four different types of collagen are known:

- Type I, the most common (found in the dermis, bone, and tendons) makes extremely strong fibrils which are highly resistant to stress.

- Type II, rich in proteoglycans, does not readily form fibrils and is mostly found in cartilaginous tissue.

- Type III, extremely rich in hydroxyproline and cysteine, this is an important type of collagen in fetal skin and, in adults, is found in association with Type I collagen in the papillary dermis, the vessels, the intestine, the uterus, and the lungs.

- Type IV is specific to the basement membrane and contains a high percentage of carbohydrates and hydroxylysine.

Each of these four types of collagen may be synthesized by different cells or the same cell may synthesize several different types (e.g., fibroblasts synthesize Types, I, II, and III).

Elastin

Elastin is a fibrous protein which is the amorphous component of elastic fibers. Its precursor is tropoelastin, which is synthesized in the endoplasmic reticulum of mesenchymal cells (fibroblasts and smooth muscle cells). Mature elastin is formed when cross-links are created between different molecules of tropoelastin. Elastin turnover is very slow and its breakdown requires specific elastase activity.

Fig. 3-7   Fascial Components

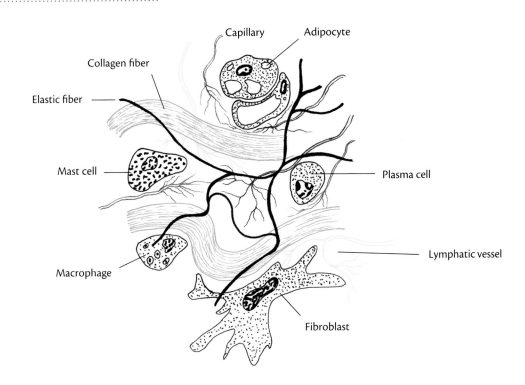

Connective tissue fibers

Three different types of fiber are found in the ground substance:

- collagen fibers
- clastic fibers
- reticular fibers

The quantity and proportions of each vary from fascia to fascia.

Collagen fibers

Collagen fibers are the most abundant in connective tissue, accounting for 60 to 70% of its overall mass. Collagen fibers are white in color, long, and completely inelastic. They are made up of bundles of parallel, unbranched fibrils, although the bundles themselves may be covalently cross-linked to one another (Fig. 3-8). The fibrils are held together by a cement substance which also coats each fiber.

In chemical terms, collagen fibers are composed of collagen, the compound which yields gelatin on boiling. It mainly consists of the amino acids glycine, praline, and hydroxyproline. Because it is completely inelastic, it confers on any tissue in which it is present both flexibility and strength.

In the early 1950's Wyckoff and Kennedy showed that collagen fibrils form a tubular structure. In 1959 Erlingheuser, theorized that these structures may circulate cerebrospinal fluid throughout the body.

Fig. 3-8 A Collagen Fiber

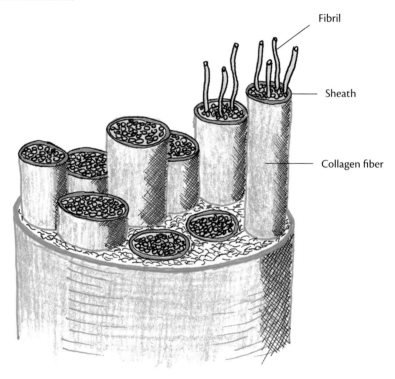

Elastic fibers

Elastic fibers are long, thin, and extensively cross-linked one to another. They can be stretched to one-and-one-half times their resting length. In chemical terms, elastin fibers are composed of elastin, an albuminoid compound which is highly resistant to heat as well as to acids and bases. Elastin fibers are yellowish in color.

The fibers are made up of an amorphous component and a microfibrillar component. With advancing age, the proportion of the amorphous component increases and the microfibrils tend to become pushed out towards the edge.

- the amorphous component is based on elastin itself
- the microfibrillar component corresponds to a structural glycoprotein

The tropoelastin from which these fibers are generated is produced by the fibroblasts of the skin and tendons, and by smooth muscle cells in the walls of major blood vessels. As is the case for collagen, the optimal temperature for the functionality of elastin is 37°C.

Reticular fibers

Reticular fibers are small collagen fibers which are found in small numbers in a microfilament-rich ground substance. They are heavily branched and are also cross-linked to one another to form a fine, extensive network. Commonly, instead of being covalently cross-linked, they simply cross over one another (Fig. 3-9).

Fig. 3-9   Reticular fibers

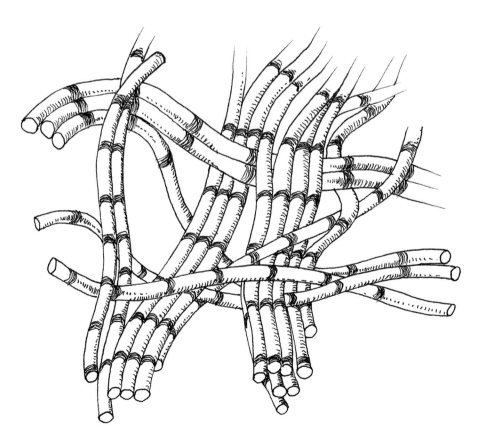

Reticular fibers are often found in basement membranes and, in continuity with collagen fibers, in lymphoid and hematopoietic tissues. They do not include ground substance. They are also found in areolar connective tissue and in adipose tissue. Fibrillar elements (collagen fibrils and fibers) may also be present.

Reticular fibers are distinct from normal collagen fibers in that they contain higher proportions of aspartic acid and hydroxyamino acids, and less proline. In addition, they are associated with a greater amount of carbohydrate.

Proteoglycans

Proteoglycans are very high molecular weight species composed of polypeptide chains to which are conjugated long polysaccharide chains called glycosamino-glycans or mucopolysaccharides. Proteoglycans bind large quantities of both water and cations, which makes them ideal for the bulk-forming function that they fulfill in the extracellular medium or ground substance of connective tissue. Their physicochemical properties are an essential factor in the viscoelastic properties of joints and other structures which are regularly subject to mechanical deformation.

Proteoglycans can act as a storage reservoir for four nutritional elements:

- carbohydrate in the form of glucose and galactose
- albumin in the form of NH groups
- lipid in hydrocarbon chains
- water, the essential component; any reduction in water content will cause retraction of the proteoglycan mass

Proteoglycans, structural glycoproteins, and the glycocalyx (a membrane which covers the external face of the cell and which mediates 'dialog' with the ground substance) are mediators and information-carrying channels. The first step in proteoglycan synthesis occurs inside the granular endoplasmic reticulum and is followed by maturation in the Golgi apparatus, and then transport out of the cell.

Different types of proteoglycan are found in different tissues:

- dermatan sulfate is mostly found in the skin, the tendons, and the walls of the arteries
- keratan sulfate occurs in the cornea, the cartilage, and the pulpy nuclei of the intervertebral disks
- hyaluronic acid is found in the more viscous body fluids (e.g., the vitreous humor and synovial fluid)

Structural glycoproteins

Structural glycoproteins play an important role in the formation of intermolecular cross-links and in orienting fibrous proteins. There seems to be a relationship between the regularity of collagen fibers and their association with glycoproteins.

In elastic lamellae, these components allow the assembly of molecules of tropoelastin.

CONNECTIVE TISSUE CELLS

Mesenchymal cells

The cytoplasm sends out processes which often give the cell a stellate morphology. These processes are often in intimate contact with neighboring cells although such adhesion points are always temporary and each cell remains independent and autonomously motile. In adult tissue, they exist as a common precursor cell which is ready to differentiate to form fibroblasts, macrophages, or the parenchymal cells of the suprarenal glands.

Fibroblasts

The fibroblast is the most common cell type in connective tissue and is present throughout life. It is these cells which produce both the ground substance and the precursors for all connective tissue fibers. They also secrete a range of enzymes involved in the catabolism of certain macromolecules and the turnover of essential structures like the basement membrane. Finally, they play a central role in the occasional processes of wound healing and inflammation.

In these cells, protocollagen is produced in the endoplasmic reticulum, matures in the Golgi apparatus, and is then transported out of the cell into the matrix. Fibroblasts also synthesize the glycosaminoglycans.

Fibroblast behavior is highly responsive to physical stimuli, so any kind of sustained tension or pressure on a fascial tissue will induce:

- local proliferation of fibroblasts
- alignment of the cells along the lines of force due to the tension or pressure
- increased secretion of macromolecules to consolidate the local fascial system in response to the stress

If stress is sustained for a long period, the fascia will become more dense and, when dissected, the tissue will be seen to be more tightly structured and its surface will present a more pearly sheen. At the same time, the way the network is organized changes according to the direction of the lines of force.

The fibroblast is the main protagonist in ground substance organization and it is the only type of cell which can coordinate the information coming from other cells and diverse nervous inputs to produce a ground substance with a composition matched to the particularities of the current situation.

The fibroblast is incapable of distinguishing between "good and bad," and, if its function is impaired, it secretes a ground substance which has structure but which is not physiologically normal. In such an abnormal environment, other cells can give rise to chronic disease processes or tumors.

Reticular cells

Reticular cells are large, star-shaped cells. Most are mesenchymal in origin, although the majority of those found in the thymus and the tonsils are probably derived from the endoderm.

Mast cells

Mast cells are immunocompetent cells which are released into connective tissue to mediate defense mechanisms. Areolar tissues are particularly rich in mast cells, particularly those in organs which contain a high concentration of heparin. They synthesize histamine, heparin, dopamine, serotonin, and hyaluronic acid, and secrete them all into the matrix.

Macrophages

Macrophages are phagocytes. While some are relatively stationary, others are highly mobile, moving between cells and fibers and ingesting any bacteria, cellular debris, or foreign matter that they encounter. They are derived from monocytes, circulating blood cells which differentiate into macrophages once they have migrated out of a vessel and arrived in the tissue.

The major role of these mobile cells is in defense mechanisms in which they participate by phagocytosing unwanted material, and secreting toxic enzymes and other biologically active species. This is the predominant cell type in both loose and dense connective tissue. Their numbers are elevated and their activity is potentiated in pathological states.

Multinucleate foreign body giant cells (which result from the fusion of macrophages and/or epithelioid cells) are found in inflammatory foci where the debris is too large to be phagocytosed by normal macrophages.

Plasma cells

Plasma cells are relatively rare in normal connective tissue, apart from in the lamina propria of the stomach wall and in the hematopoietic organs. However, they are present in great numbers in chronically inflamed connective tissue (e.g., in the gastrointestinal tract, the lymph nodes, or the spleen). These are the cells which are responsible for producing antibodies.

Leukocytes

Leukocytes—lymphocytes, monocytes, and polymorphonuclear cells—migrate out of the circulation into the tissues. They are mobilized to mediate inflammatory responses and defend against attacking pathogens.

Adipocytes

Adipocytes are found in the collagen fiber network in all kinds of tissue, either on their own or in clusters. In certain areas, like around the kidney or the suprarenal gland, they are constantly in a cycle of growth and turnover. In adults, most adipocytes are found in white adipose tissue, although another form, brown adipose tissue, is predominant in new-borns.

The main function of these cells is fat storage. This can serve a variety of purposes:

- the first and most important reason for storing fats is to have a reserve of neutral lipid (created by the process of lipogenesis) which can be released into the circulation (lipolysis) when extra energy is required
- a layer of lipid also acts as an efficient thermal insulator
- fatty tissue is also important in terms of mechanical protection in that it attenuates pressure and acts as a shock absorber

Pigment cells

Various cells synthesize and store different types of pigment with specific chemical natures and particular colors. The most widely known is melanin, a dark brown or black pigment which is found in melanocytes.

VARIOUS TYPES OF CONNECTIVE TISSUE

Mesenchyma

Mesenchymal tissue is found in the embryo and is characterized by a ground substance with a high water content and which contains no fibers.

Wharton's jelly

Wharton's jelly is a soft, homogenous intercellular substance which is found in the umbilical cord. It contains fewer cells than mesenchyma but its ground substance is more viscous and it contains a few fibers. It is never found in adults apart from certain pathological conditions (e.g., in patients with papilloma or myxoma).

Reticular tissue

Reticular tissue is the most primitive form of connective tissue found in adults. It is made up of reticular cells and very fine, silver-staining fibers. Some of the cells are bound to the fibers, others are unbound. This type of tissue is found in:

- lymph nodes
- spleen and liver
- bone marrow

Areolar connective tissue

This is based on a loose network of collagen, elastic, and reticular fibers in a rich, soft ground substance. All the cells which are found in other types of adult connective tissue are also present in areolar connective tissue, apart from reticular cells.

Any exchange process between the blood vessels and the parenchyma of organs necessarily involves passage through this medium, which makes it important in cellular nutrition. This type of connective tissue in the submucosa is a key factor in the motility of the gastrointestinal tract.

The mechanical properties of areolar connective tissue are plasticity and elasticity, both of which are largely due to the consistency of the ground substance. Within this tissue are found immunocompetent cells, blood vessels, and nerves. It forms the stroma of most of the solid organs where it functions as a kind of packing material in the:

- gastrointestinal submucosa
- mucosa of the airways and genitourinary tract
- cutaneous dermis
- submesothelial layer of serous membranes

It is part of the make-up of peripheral nerves and muscles, and is also found in both superficial and deep fasciae.

Adipose tissue

Adipose tissue is a special type of connective tissue which is highly vascular and rich in adipocytes. It is particularly abundant in certain areas like the kidneys, the ischioanal fossa, the omentum, the subcutaneous tissue, and the mesentery.

In embryogenesis, spherical capillary plexi develop in these areas even before any fat has been deposited. A lobule of adipose tissue grows in the territory of such a plexus until neighboring lobules come into contact with one another, although they remain separated by fibrous septa. In subcutaneous tissue, such septa are called cutaneous ligaments. These lobules of adipose tissue act as cushions to absorb excess pressure as well as serving as fat storage depots.

Two different types of adipose tissue exist, white fat and brown fat. In human adults, almost all of the adipose tissue is white. Brown adipose tissue predominates in new-borns.

Dense connective tissue

Dense connective tissue is full of fibers and, being exceptionally strong, plays a key mechanical role. It contains few blood vessels but dense networks of collagen and elastic fibers.

Distinction is usually made between two different types of dense connective tissue:

- irregular
- regular

Irregular dense connective tissue

Irregular dense connective tissue resembles areolar connective tissue, but contains a denser network of thicker collagen fibers which makes it firmer and stronger (Fig. 3-10). It is found in the dermis, the capsules of certain organs, the dura mater, the deep fasciae, the periosteum, the perichondrium, cartilage, and bone.

Fig. 3-10 Dense, Irregular Connective Tissue

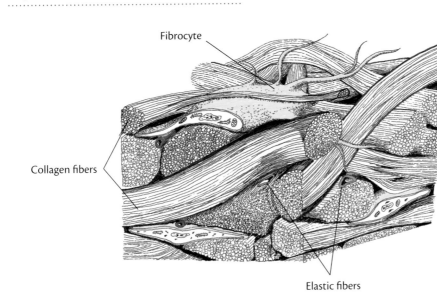

Fibrocyte

Collagen fibers

Elastic fibers

Regular dense connective tissue

This type of dense connective tissue is found in the tendons, the aponeuroses, the ligaments, and the stroma of the cornea. Tendons are made up of thick collagen fibers which are tightly bundled together in a parallel arrangement.

These bundles are separated from one another by sheets of areolar connective tissue, and the entire structure is invested by a fibrous sheath composed of more dense connective tissue (Fig. 3-11).

Aponeuroses are composed of sheets of fibers arranged in parallel, with alternating sheets disposed at right angles to one another. Fasciae (which can be considered as resulting from the coming together of aponeuroses) have the same basic structure.

From a histological point of view, ligaments resemble tendons. Elastic ligaments (ligamenta flava) contain, in addition, bundles of thick elastic fibers arranged in parallel and separated by small amounts of areolar connective tissue. Fibroblasts tend to be more sparse in this type of fiber.

Fig. 3-11 Arterial Connective Tissue

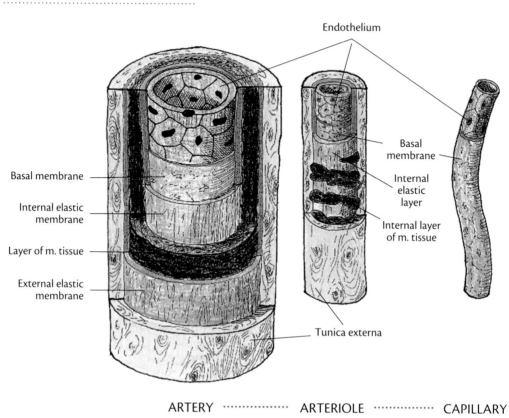

ARTERY ·················· ARTERIOLE ··············· CAPILLARY

4

Fascial Pathology

CONNECTIVE TISSUE, AS discussed above, is found in all compartments of the body. As all the various tissues are in intimate contact with one another, it seems obvious that whichever particular part of the body has some dysfunction or disease, to some extent connective tissue will necessarily and automatically be involved. Regardless of whether a given health problem is neurological, rheumatologic, cardiovascular or gastrointestinal, it is clear that any abnormality with all its particularities will be reflected in the status of the connective tissue. It is generally believed that problems in connective tissue diffuse distally via the nervous system.

Connective tissue and collagen diseases are classified as specific diseases in textbooks of pathology, but all such conditions share a common characteristic, namely, degeneration of the ground substance of the connective tissue. The surprising phenomenon is the far-ranging nature of these diseases, which usually involve multiple systems. However, is this really so surprising in view of the ubiquity of connective tissue?

These two types of disease also share certain other features:

- the clinical symptoms of inflammatory diseases
- poor prognosis for total recovery
- non-specific symptoms and frequently atypical clinical pictures which render diagnosis difficult

Damaged connective tissue takes time to recover, a process that cannot be rushed. The return to a normal state within the actual connective tissue itself may take two to three years. There is no possibility for regulation if the connective tissue is mechanically paralyzed, as is seen in progressive, chronic, degenerative processes.

Collagen Diseases

FOUR MAJOR COLLAGEN DISEASES

There are four major collagen diseases that are relatively prevalent at present:

- systemic lupus erythematosus
- scleroderma
- polyarteritis nodosa
- ermatomyositis

We will not analyze or even describe these diseases in any detail, but rather merely note that there is a great degree of overlap among their many and diverse symptoms. These diseases can involve just about any part of the body, but primarily affect the:

- skin
- muscles
- joints
- chest
- nervous system
- internal organs

The more or less intense involvement of multiple systems in collagen disease underlines the importance of the connective tissue, which is distributed throughout all parts of the body. As an example, consider the cutaneous manifestations of just one of these diseases, schleroderma. This provides a good illustration of how connective tissue problems can cause pathology. Scleroderma is characterized by excessive accumulation of collagen. In patients with this condition, atrophied, thin epidermis ends up covering a compact mass of collagen fibers that run parallel to the epidermis. Fingerlike projections of collagen extend down from the dermis into the subcutaneous tissue and bind the skin to the deeper layers of tissue.

OTHER MAJOR COLLAGEN DISEASES

There are other significant diseases that affect the connective tissues. Some of the major ones include:

Wegener's granulomatosis

An autoimmune vasculitis which is characterized by severe involvement of the upper respiratory tract, the lungs and kidneys.

Mixed connective tissue disease

The most common overlap being rheumatic disease syndrome, which is characterized by a combination of clinical features relating to systemic lupus erythematosus, scleroderma, and other collagen diseases.

Marfan's syndrome

A disorder in which certain parts of the connective tissue are weakened. It is characterized by excessive height, abnormally long limbs, especially at the extremities, reduced vision due to dislocation of the lenses, arachnodactyly, overly lax joints, and some visceral abnormalities such as aortic aneurysms.

Rheumatoid arthritis

Now classified as a collagen disease. It is characterized at the tissue level by synovitis, vasculitis, and rheumatoid nodules. Rheumatoid nodules are usually subcutaneous and are most common around pressure points, such as the elbows. Similar nodules may occur in the pleura, the lungs, and the heart, and, rarely, in the capsule of the liver or the vocal cords. The nodule consists of an inner zone of fibrinoid necrosis surrounded by a cuff of macrophages that is, in turn, surrounded by a layer of fibrous connective tissue containing large numbers of lymphocytes and plasma cells.

Other Diseases of the Fasciae

In addition to the specific collagen diseases mentioned above, there are other abnormalities that involve connective tissue which do not usually present as dramatic a clinical picture, but are certainly more common.

First, we shall discuss scars and adhesions. These abnormalities and non-functionalities are of special interest to osteopaths because they are so frequently encountered in their daily practice. Furthermore, in the long term, scars and adhesions can act as foci of irritation that can, in turn, interfere with the functioning of the joints and viscera. This initially leads to the type of symptom which is referred to as functional, since such manifestations are often subclinical and do not correspond to any abnormality that can be detected in conventional radiological or biochemical tests.

Scars and adhesions are genuine primary lesions that must be examined with the greatest care.

Later we shall discuss different studies of the connective tissues, in particular those focusing on its ground substance, that tend to show that the disease process often arises in the matrix, especially when it has become overwhelmed by exogenous factors.

We will make reference to the work of Snyder, who in 1956 proposed that the ground substance is both the laboratory of the connective tissue and a propitious terrain for the development of pathological processes.

SCARS

Wound healing involves tissue remodeling with granulation and the proliferation of elastic and connective fibers. The ultimate aim of this process is to regenerate as nearly as possible the tissue's original structure. Notwithstanding the sophistication of the repair mechanisms, they cannot always be perfect; the traces left by any scar which impinges on the deep fasciae serve as an example. While in most cases the repair is made without any consequences, in a significant proportion of cases the resultant scar can disrupt the functioning of the surrounding tissues. This can manifest as irritation which may, in turn, lead to restrictions or even frank adhesions which interfere with both mechanical and physiological function. Excluding retractile scars and keloids, both of which are relatively rare, even an ordinary scar may end up causing pathology. This can have very serious consequences for the patient, as in cases of causalgia. In particular, a pruritic scar may perturb connective tissue and lead to changes in its structure, plasticity, and elasticity secondary to the concomitant tension and stress at the focus of irritation. Sooner or later, this will lead to mechanical disturbance of the fasciae over a more or less extensive area.

When the scar is in the abdominal region—the most common site due to the large number of appendectomies that are performed—it will interfere with the mechanics of the neighboring organs, subjecting them to tension and constant irritation. The organ will tend to lose its mobility and become fixed. We have already seen that normal physiological function depends on fascial mobility; therefore. such immobilization of an organ will lead to dysfunction and, in the long term, disease.

Scar tissue can also become pathological as a result of foreign bodies which became trapped at the time of the injury. Foreign bodies are only reabsorbed slowly, if at all, and when they persist, they can induce acidosis in surrounding tissues which compromises the composition and function of the local ground substance.

Electrical measurements made in 'disturbed' scar tissue show that its resistance is of the order of 1,400 kilo-ohms higher than that of surrounding normal skin.

For all of these reasons a scar must be considered as a potential source of problems.

ADHESIONS

Adhesions are a common problem and may result from scarring, inflammation and infection, irritation, or any kind of increase in stress anywhere in the body. They are particularly common in the thorax and abdomen. Simple incision into the peritoneum is quite likely to trigger some kind of adhesion. The tendency to form adhesions increases with age and a surprisingly high number of adhesions are routinely observed in the pleura, the lungs, and the peritoneum at autopsy.

The sequelae of adhesions are similar to those of scars in that they often lead to the formation of solid, inelastic, fibrous connections to an organ. We shall return later to the vicious circle of hypomobility, dysfunction, and disease.

DUPUYTREN'S CONTRACTURE

In the context of connective tissue disease, mention should also be made of Dupuytren's contracture. This is a condition characterized by thickening and retraction of the middle palmar aponeurosis. The etiology of this highly specific and localized fascial problem is unknown.

CONNECTIVE TISSUE, THE POINT OF DEPARTURE FOR MANY DISEASE PROCESSES

Studies of the histology and the role of connective tissue have shown that any kind of injury, shock, or stress automatically has an effect on the local connective tissue. We may conclude that there is no pathology that does not have any impact on the fasciae. In fact, no disease process can spread until it has overcome the defensive capacities of connective tissue.

Eppinger (noted in Pischinger) has postulated that disease starts in the ground substance and spreads from there to parenchymatous cells. Specific symptoms and the typical characteristics of the disease take form only later, after cellular lesions have developed—distinctly later than the prodromal symptoms of the various infectious entities.

Connective tissue can be irritated by many different factors, in fact, by any situation that involves stress being put on the fasciae, for example, physical injury, mechanical stress, chemical insults, and endocrine effects. Postoperative shock is a prime example: the body takes approximately 21 days to recover from the shock of surgery.

The ground substance is not only the starting point for messages destined for the cell and the endocrine and nervous systems, but is also itself modified when tissue function is impaired. Even very mild stimulation of short duration induces partial depolarization of proteoglycan molecules. In a normally functioning system, this depolarization is compensated for by a charge of opposing polarity. However, if such stimulation and depolarization is sustained, structural changes can occur in the ground substance which result in a marked increase in its viscosity such that it becomes more gel-like in consistency. Such changes remain localized at first, since the spread of information is limited by the insulating properties of the serous membranes, the septa, and the fasciae.

At first it is difficult to detect disturbances in the connective tissues, all the more so since such disturbances do not usually give rise to symptoms which are typical of irritation. As a result, the tissues can often continue transmitting an abnormal signal for a relatively long time, thereby misleading the regulatory cellular, tissue, endocrine, and nervous systems for a prolonged period. Changes in regulatory processes spread out gradually, and the symptoms can spread to the opposite side of the body with the indirect participation of the vertebral axis. Any additional stimulation of this primed system will frequently lead to an inappropriate and exaggerated response.

Remote problems (e.g., in an organ) may occur, increasing even further the irritation at the original focus and leading eventually, in the absence of intervention, to exhaustion and to a reactional block which can result in serious disease. Perger (noted in Pischinger) points out that 25% of patients presenting with a "block of basic regulation" developed a tumor in the years that followed. The role of regulatory problems in the etiology of tumor development cannot be neglected.

Furthermore, both an active potential and increased conductivity have been observed on the same side of the body as the pathology in chronically sick individuals.

The damage is localized at first in the dermatome and the myotome, but through the action of the autonomic nervous system, the injury modifies local vasomotor functions as well as other autonomous functions in the entire corresponding quadrant. Any increase in the intensity of stimulation, or any kind of activation of central regulatory mechanisms, will lead to the development of symptoms in the whole area surrounding the focus of primary damage.

Following on from the local problems, systemic disease can develop if secondary and tertiary factors come into play. The connective tissue then reacts as a unit, though not necessarily in the same way in all places. Differences are all the more pronounced if the rate of progress of the chronic problem has accelerated. The timing and duration of the original insult have a major impact in terms of how the disturbance spreads around the body as a whole.

Certain mesenchymal cells in adult connective tissue remain at an immature stage of development and these embryonic-type stem cells can, in case of need, differentiate into other lineages of more specialized cells. As a rule, these cells are in a dormant state but, in case of injury or disease, they can undergo mitotic proliferation to help manage the effects of the insult.

It appears that the activation of defense mechanisms in connective tissue occurs independently in the periphery, with the central system only intervening at a later stage. This is born out by the observations that both the highest baseline measurements and the most severe damage are always found on the side of the body that is most severely perturbed. Damaged tissue (from inflammation, scarring, adhesions, etc.) that cannot be reabsorbed is responsible for such differences between the two sides of the body.

Two other researchers discussed in Pischinger's excellent book add to this concept. Kellner has demonstrated that the body's acid–base balance is determined by a fundamental homeostatic mechanism: when the milieu is acidic, neutral pH is re-established by the lysis of fibroblasts, but when the milieu is alkaline, the same cells proliferate. McLaughlin found that embryonic epithelial cells cultured in vitro tended to grow in an undifferentiated and disorganized way. The addition of mesenchymal cells induced differentiation of the epithelial cells. Moreover, in the presence of these other cells, a basement membrane was formed and the cells formed a stratified pattern. These two experiments tend to show that connective tissue comprises a self-organizing system which does not depend to central control mechanisms.

In response to persistent stress, functional difficulties arise and the activity of the ground substance in terms of its role as a molecular filter is compromised. This can lead to changes in ground substance composition and, therefore, to enhanced susceptibility to chronic disease.

Heine (discussed in Pischinger) has shown that 30 minutes suffice to stimulate a significant increase in collagen content in the alveolar septa of badly injured traffic accident victims. Speransky (noted in Korr) performed experiments in animals which demonstrated that profound modifications of lung tissue (similar to those seen in pneumonia) could be brought about by various modes of nervous stimulation, including intense stimulation of cutaneous and muscular receptors in the area innervated from the medulla oblongata or the upper part of the spinal cord. Mechanical or direct chemical stimulation of the nerve center was observed to have similar effects.

Thus, it appears that connective tissue has some degree of autonomy and that it may have its own, independent defense systems. It also represents the point of departure of many pathological processes, a point of departure which is itself independent. This mechanism does not exclude the possibility that peripheral or central stimulation of the afferent nerves may also lead to perturbation of connective tissue. This point has to be kept in mind when diagnosing any kind of disruption or disease in any part of the body.

5

The Roles of the Fasciae

AS WE HAVE seen, the fasciae fulfill many different roles in the body, and the unique adaptability of their basic structure equips them for these different functions.

The fasciae, and by extension connective tissues in general, are found throughout the body. The results of anatomical and physiological studies lead to the conclusion that connective tissue plays a major role in the maintenance of all body functions. Different studies dealing with the subject show that the connective tissue provides the ultimate guarantee for the proper functioning of the body, and thus for its health. As George Snyder stated back in 1956, "the connective tissues not only bind the various parts of the body, but, in a broader sense, connect the numerous branches of medicine."

The different roles of the fasciae will be studied in the following order:

- in maintaining structural integrity
- in support
- in protection
- as shock absorbers
- in hemodynamic processes
- in defense
- in communication and exchange processes
- in biochemical processes

A continuous network of connective tissue links all the different organs and parts of the body. Anatomical studies have shown that there is no discontinuity between the different tissues, but that they are linked together to function in perfect harmony (Fig. 5-1).

Fig. 5-1 Fascial Support

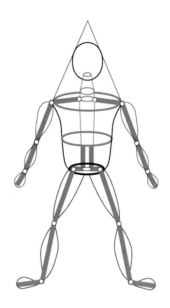

Role in maintaining structural integrity

The fasciae maintain the anatomical integrity of the individual. A person would retain a perfectly human appearance even if one removed all the body systems but the fasciae. The same would be true if one attempted to retain only the vascular or nervous system, as the fasciae provide the supporting and guiding structures for both of these systems. This confirms once again the interdependence of the different structures of the body and the impossibility of dissociating them.

The muscular system only functions by virtue of the fasciae, as we shall see when we consider the mechanics of this system of tissues. Moreover, it is because of the fasciae that the joints can maintain their stability and function. The muscular system constitutes the motor of the joints, but the coordination of that system is completely dependent on the mechanical properties of the fasciae.

Different organs maintain their shape and are attached to the bones by virtue of the fasciae. The fasciae thus maintain the anatomical integrity of the organs and thereby make it possible for them to function correctly.

Role in support

The fasciae support the nervous, arterial, venous, and lymphatic systems. Anatomical studies show that these different systems are intimately linked to the fasciae. Indeed, these systems are themselves constituted of fasciae, which maintain their shape and form. Furthermore, they are surrounded by a fascial envelope that, in turn, is linked to and shaped by denser, stronger fascial elements.

The nervous and vascular systems interact with the fascial system. During embryonic development, the vascular and nervous systems grow and migrate together with the fasciae in a parallel, coordinated series of steps.

The supporting role becomes particularly evident at the level of the deep cervical fascia: these cannot be separated from the cervical plexus or the sympathetic cervical ganglions. A similar picture is seen in the mesenteries, which support an abundance of different vessels and nerves.

Role in protection

The fasciae play a fundamental role in maintaining the physical and physiological integrity of the human body. Present throughout the body, they protect the different anatomical structures against the varied and potentially dangerous forces of tension and stress to which the body is constantly exposed. In fulfilling this role, the fasciae of the different body compartments show an impressive degree of adaptability and variation.

In the periphery, where potentially damaging forces are greatest, the fasciae tend to be thicker and denser. In and around the joints, the fasciae which form the synovial membranes and, to an even greater extent, those which constitute the ligaments, are extremely strong and stable. Although these fasciae are strong, they are never rigid; complete rigidity is only found in pathological situations, and functional fasciae always retain some degree of elasticity, enough to fulfill their role in the specific tissue in which they are found.

When the work load is heavy, thickened fasciae can completely replace muscle bundles. The most typical examples of this phenomenon are the powerful iliotibial tract and the highly resistant lumbosacral aponeurosis.

Another protective role, as we shall see in more detail later, consists of the ability of the fasciae to act as shock absorbers. In response to over-exertion or to forces which are too violent, the fasciae absorb some of the energy of the excessive shock so as to protect muscles, organs, and other structures from damage. Such intervention is triggered by stimulation of the nerve endings in fascial tissue. It has been demonstrated that while the anterior longitudinal ligament has a passive function, it is richly innervated. It shows strong neurological activity when stimulated (Bednar, 1995).

Throughout the entire length of the cerebrospinal axis, the fasciae protect the brain and spinal cord against excessive variations in pressure as well as potentially damaging shocks. The fasciae in these tissues are remarkably adaptable and ingenious. A single connective tissue envelope would be insufficient to protect such delicate structures; thus, a triple envelope of fascial sheets has evolved, and, in order to further enhance the efficacy of the system, two hydraulic buffering systems have been added in the form of the cerebrospinal fluid and a dense network of veins.

The protective role of the fasciae is also key in the vascular and nervous systems that the fasciae not only support, but also protect from compression, stretching, and other insults.

It may be recalled that the major arteriovenous and nerve trunks are found in the deep fasciae and that the latter are either sheathed in fascial envelopes (e.g., the adductor canal) or are located in the most stable parts of the fasciae (e.g., the root of the mesentery).

Finally, to protect vital and fragile organs, the fasciae not only invest them with a resistant sheath, but also cushion them with an additional layer of tissue. This cushioning layer can be based on either a very fluid and plastic form of tissue, such as adipose tissue (e.g., the adipose cushion around the kidney), or a very loosely woven tissue, such as areolar tissue.

The organs themselves have a fascial envelope that maintains their structure. Extensions from the envelope penetrate into the interior of the organ where they split frequently to divide the organ into a series of different compartments, with the contents of each isolated to a greater or lesser extent from those of its neighbors. One consequence is that it limits the rate of spread of infection from one part of an organ to another. The clearest examples of this kind of compartmentalization are to be found in the liver and the lungs.

Role of shock absorber

The elastic fasciae often act to dampen the forces to which the body is subject. The lattice-like macromolecular structure of the proteoglycans participates actively in the mechanical cohesiveness of connective tissue.

The proteoglycans are shock absorbers that act like lubricants which, under intense, repeated stress, change texture to become more viscoelastic. The proteoglycans and hyaluronic acid impose a cross-linked molecular superstructure upon the ground substance and invest and fill the spaces between collagen and elastic fibers; this viscoelastic buffering material is indispensable for the normal functioning of cells and tissues. The work of Yahia, et al. (1993) confirms this; they investigated the viscoelastic behavior of the lumbodorsal fasciae and found that it steadily changed over time in response to repeated challenges with a heavy load.

Furthermore, the fasciae attenuate the effects of high pressure by channeling the energy in different directions to prevent damage to the organs. Fascial shock absorber function is potentiated by the adipose tissue, which is particularly abundant in certain vulnerable regions, for example, around the kidney, over the abdomen, and over the greater omentum. Similar accumulations of adipose tissue are found in regions which are subject to particularly high levels of pressure, such as around the ischiorectal fossa.

An aside is appropriate here on the shock absorber function of the meninges. We have seen that these structures line the skull as well as the spinal column and protect the cerebrospinal axis. However, the meninges also contain the cerebrospinal fluid, and thereby act as a fluid envelope that serves as shock absorber for the brain, protecting it against any variation in pressure to which it is exposed. The fluid also has a nutritional and defensive role. Most of the fluid is secreted by the choroid plexus with approximately 20% coming directly from the venous parenchyma in the Virchow-Robin perivascular spaces. The fluid is reabsorbed both by the veins via the villi and Pacchioni's arachnoid granulations, and by the lymphatics in the neural sheath. Then it is transferred into the thoracic canal.

In the adult, the volume of cerebrospinal fluid is 140ml ± 30ml, of which 35ml are in the ventricles, 25ml in the cerebral subarachnoid spaces and cisterns, and 75ml in the spinal subarachnoids. Its qualitative composition resembles that of plasma and lymph, but the various components are in different proportions. It also contains a number of hormones and other substances whose role is not yet clear. New cerebral substances are being discovered constantly and this research is furthering our understanding of the role of the cerebrospinal fluid. The most recent instance is a substance with strong soporific activity discovered by Richard Lerner (Huidobro-Toro and Harris, 1996).

Cerebrospinal fluid is produced at the rate of 0.5–1.0 l per 24 hours. Fluctuations in the volume of the cerebrospinal fluid due to expansion and retraction of the system constitute one of the driving forces of the cranial mechanism which has a frequency of 8–12 cycles per second. In fact, it appears that this rhythm of 8–12 cycles per second is probably more characteristic of a 'pathological' state due to a kind of sympathicotonia, which is related to the stress of modern life. The cranial rhythm in primitive societies is approximately 2.5 periods per minute, which leads us to believe that this frequency more closely corresponds to the natural, equilibrium state.

Observation of these rhythmic movements of the brain and fluctuations in the volume of the cerebrospinal fluid have given rise to a hypothesis according to which it is the circulation of the cerebrospinal fluid through the fasciae which is causing these rhythmic movements. It appears, however, that there is no continuity between the cerebrospinal fluid and the peripheral tissues, particularly at the level of the nerve roots.

Rydevick et al. injected [^{3}H]methylglucose, either intravenously or directly into the cerebrospinal fluid and found the following distributions of isotopes:

- after injection into a nerve root, 58% in the cerebrospinal fluid versus 35% in the intramural vessels
- after injection into a peripheral nerve, 95% in the intramural vessels and none in cerebrospinal fluid

Most of the nutritional requirements of the nerve roots are supplied by the cerebrospinal fluid whereas those of the peripheral nerves come almost exclusively from the blood. There is no evidence that any cerebrospinal fluid ever reaches the peripheral nerves.

The cranial and spinal nerves beyond the osseous openings are invested by connective tissue through which lymph circulates.

The meninges thus have a close relationship with the lymph spaces; there is no direct continuity, but these two contiguous systems participate in multiple exchange processes. This is altogether logical since, if there were continuity between the cerebrospinal fluid and the periphery, there would be a major risk of the spread of infection to the brain (since there are so many ports of entry for foreign microorganisms in the periphery). The fact that exchanges occur exclusively by diffusion constitutes a safety buffer comparable to those found in many other regions of the body. Therefore, the cerebrospinal fluid communicates with the extracellular fluid in the same way as the latter communicates with the intracellular fluid.

Throughout the system, communication is by diffusion or active transport, but never direct. The different fluids differ in chemical composition but are in permanent contact, assuring continuity and communication through the entire the body.

Role in hemodynamic processes

The vascular and lymphatic systems cannot be dissociated from the fascial system. The return circulation in the form of the venous and lymphatic systems does not include any active pump as powerful as that which sends the blood to all parts of the body via the arteries. Furthermore, the latter have a rigid structure, unlike the lymphatics and the veins, which are relatively flaccid and collapse readily. For this reason, these vessels are equipped with valves to facilitate the return of blood and lymph, although they cannot perform this function without help.

It is actually the fasciae that provide the pumping force for the return circulation of blood and lymph. As we shall see, the fasciae are continually pulsing with a frequency of about 8 to 12 cycles per minute. These contractions act as a pump which drives the fluids through the vessels.

It should be noted that the transport of lymph through the lymphatics depends on sequential contractions of the valvular segments. The lymph is transported by waves of contraction with a frequency of 10 to 12 cycles per minute. This is equivalent to the period of the fasciae—but of course the lymphatic system is primarily composed of fascial elements.

This subtle mechanism is reinforced by muscular contractions which are also channeled by the fasciae. Anatomy shows us that the fasciae are not continuous parallel bands, but rather are constituted of different layers arranged in oblique, transverse, and circular orientations. The different orientations of the fascial fibers mean that the overall configuration of the fasciae corresponds to a spiral arrangement. Hence, when they contract, they have a tendency to compress the structures that they are investing, thereby pushing the fluids back towards the heart, just like a dishcloth that is being wrung out.

However, if the fasciae are the motor of the return circulation, they can also be a disrupting element: if a fascia is in a state of abnormal tension, it is easy to understand that the associated vascular system will be subject to sustained pressure, which will induce stasis.

The lymphatics and veins perforate the fasciae through more or less rigid ring structures that let the tubes traverse the fasciae without encumbrance. However, if any of these annular openings is ever put under great tension, it can be converted into a tourniquet.

Role in defense

The ultimate function of the connective tissue is to re-establish normal defense functions. Their defensive role is certainly a major aspect of the physiology of the fasciae. The fight against pathogenic agents and infections starts in the ground substance in which there is an intrinsic local mechanism which is active prior to any kind of intervention on the part of the specialized immune system. Whether or not the pathogenic agent has time to spread—and hence the health of the subject—depends on this local mechanism.

The process of defense is characterized by four cellular phases:

- at the beginning, the site of invasion is walled off by macrophages
- this is followed immediately by attack by smaller phagocytic cells—microphages (a local reaction, but with the passive participation of the whole body)
- subsequently, there is a macrophage phase with the active participation of the whole body
- the final stage involves specialized lymphocytes (leading to sterilization of the infection and establishment of a chronic state)

The macrophage phase is triggered by a monocyte factor, and in the absence of this factor, there is no such phase.

The first local defense reactions are triggered when a series of signaling molecules is released into the tissue (prostaglandins, leukotrienes, interferon, etc.) The triggering of the macrophage and microphage phases does not only depend on biochemical factors, but also on biophysical ones like the abrupt drop in pH at the site of injury. This acidosis can damage cell membranes. Conversely, major biophysical changes at the site of injury can set in motion an immediate emergency reaction that triggers a primary defense response to limit the extent of the damage. This occurs in two phases:

- Disruption of the bonds which are keeping the large reticular cells confined in the basal system. Their release as macrophages results in the isolation of the site of invasion.
- Modification of the permeability of the capillary walls, which results in the onset of the microphage phase.

These phenomena are accompanied by the extravasation of serum into the tissues, which leads to edema. This edema is not detrimental to the efficacy of the defense system, as was believed at one time; on the contrary, it may even dilute the noxious agent. The extravasation of serum also means that, if the specific microorganism has been encountered before, any anamnestic serum globulins are recruited to act at the site of attack.

This defense mechanism, as pointed out earlier, starts at the level of the ground substance. The ground substance is linked to the endocrine glands by capillaries, and to the central nervous system by the free terminal ends of autonomic and other nerves. Both of these organizing systems are located in the cerebral trunk. The ground substance can thus exert a direct influence on the higher regulatory centers when certain species (interleukins, prostaglandins, interferon, proteases, etc.) are released into it. There is exchange of information between the capillaries, the autonomic nerve fibers, and the motile cells of the ground substance (macrophages, leukocytes, and monocytes). The result is an endocrine network of extraordinary complexity and sophistication.

The advantage of network-based systems is enhanced adaptability and efficiency. The aim of the body is to maintain a constant internal milieu by means of homeostatic regulation.

In phylogenetic terms, the ground substance is more ancient than either the nervous or the endocrine system. As a result, the generation and turnover of ground substance is governed by a primitive compensatory cellular organizational system based on the synergistic action of fibroblasts and macrophages. Fibroblasts can react within seconds by synthesizing the appropriate proteoglycans and structural glycoproteins in the quantities required. These are destined to be phagocytosed by the macrophages. As the quality of the ground substance becomes progressively more compromised, the fibroblast begins to secrete a kind of ground substance which has structure, but which is not fully functional. When exposed to this defective ground substance for extended periods of time, any cell can, according to Heine, become pathological or malignant (Pischinger, 1991).

Other substances are also important in terms of the defensive function of the ground substance. The proteoglycans and glycosaminoglycans constitute the first system of defense; being highly viscoelastic, they absorb shocks, resulting in the dissipation of energy.

Selye (as noted in Pischinger) considered connective tissue to be the regulator of the stress syndrome. The stress syndrome leads to premature aging as a result of a lack of adaptability, largely due to the loss of the energy required for adaptation. This defensive role of connective tissue is illustrated by the functions of the peritoneum and of the greater omentum. The major functions of the peritoneum are to reduce friction, to store fat (in the greater omentum), and to resist infection. The greater omentum tends to orient itself towards the site of infection (by mechanisms which are as yet poorly understood), and to move closer to the site, thereby increasing the local blood supply. In this manner, it helps prevent the spread of infection.

It appears, on the basis of our current knowledge, that only at relatively late stages do the specialized cells of the immune system play an active role in fighting infections. The ground substance appears to represent the first defensive barrier.

Role in communication and exchange processes

The connective tissue, and especially the ground substance, are in contact with the cells of the body. The vascular, lymphatic, and nervous systems terminate in the ground substance and do not extend beyond the level of the cell. All of these different systems provide nutrients to the ground substance and carry information from the periphery. Similarly, they remove the waste products of metabolism and take back information from the cells.

The cells are bathed in extracellular fluid, and a dialog occurs with the ground substance via that fluid. The function of the ground substance is, as we have seen, to provide a defensive barrier to protect the cells from damage.

Once the ground substance has been overwhelmed by a pathogenic agent, the cell itself may be affected and degeneration and morbidity may ensue. In addition to its defensive role, the ground substance is in permanent contact with the cell, furnishing it with the products that it needs for its functioning as well as transporting in the opposite direction the products of cellular metabolism and messages.

The connective tissue is considered to be a unitary complex that invests specialized parenchymatous cells and helps them to survive, as well as regulating some of their key functions.

As noted in Pischinger, as early as 1767, Bordeu understood that connective tissue was there not only for padding and support, but also for the regulation and nutrition of the organs. He also recognized its importance in vascular and nervous function.

Connective tissue is an element which links the parenchyma with the vascular and nervous systems. Exchanges with cells occur by diffusion, osmosis, and active processes across the serous membranes (Fig. 5-2)

Fig. 5-2   Exchange Processes Between Cells and Fasciae

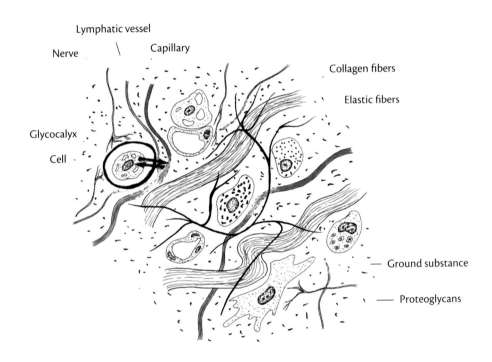

The carbohydrate-rich surface film of the cell, the glycocalyx, is the functional intermediary between the intracellular environment and the extracellular space. It communicates with the receptive cell envelope via glycosaminoglycans and proteoglycans, and establishes contact between the intracellular milieu and the ground substance. Perturbations of the latter may alter the carbohydrate composition of the glycocalyx and thereby modify the behavior of the cell.

There are also binding proteins such as fibronectin, laminin, and chondronectin which act as intermediaries between the cell surface and the ground substance.

Fibronectin is important in growth, mobility, and cell differentiation, and participates in the binding of the cells to the ground substance, and therefore in the superimposition of different layers of cells. Tenascin, a recently discovered glycoprotein, is believed to be important in interactions between different cells.

Heparin, found in the vesicles of mast cells and basophils, is released when it is needed. It participates in all aspects of the regulation of the ground substance:

- it regulates lipolysis and the levels of lipoproteins in the blood
- it stimulates the aggregation of lymphoid cells
- it activates the protein kinases of muscle cells
- it stimulates synthesis of the ground substance, and participates in the synthesis of collagen and its polymerization to form fibrils

Basement membranes are made of a special form of ground substance. They are indispensable for the normal epithelial growth and also invest Schwann cells, terminal axons, striated and smooth muscle cells, and the cells of the myocardium. Changes in basement membrane structure can have serious consequences for the integrity and function of organs.

Basement membranes block the spread of inflammatory processes from the connective tissue to the epithelium. This activity seems to be due to the high concentration of vitamin C in these structures which traps, detoxifies, and therefore blocks the passage of the free radicals generated in inflammatory reactions.

The parenchyma is nourished via a secretory current which flows across the capillary membranes towards the plasma membrane where the metabolite-rich fluid is available for the parenchymatous cells. At that point, this fluid comes into contact with the extremely dense network of lymphatics that runs through connective tissue.

Role in biochemical processes

Following the research work of Philippe Bourdinaud (inspired by the work of Dan Urry, a chemical engineer at the University of Minnesota) on the biochemical action of the osteopath's hand on human connective tissue, we now know that the elastin, reticular, and collagen fibers (all bioplymers) found in the fascial matrix are able to retract under the influence of pressure higher than the physiological pressure for which their biochemical composition fits them. When the pressure of the interstitial milieu returns to normal, they in turn return to their normal length.

The phenomenon of retraction occurs because, under the influence of high pressure, water molecules in the fascial matrix reorganize to form cage-like structures around the hydrophobic ends of the fibers. The reverse transition is also possible, that is, they can return to their original length if the pressure in the fascial matrix is released or returns to a normal physiological level. This occurs through the formation of hydrogen bonds between the water molecules and the fascial matrix and the hydrophilic ends of the fibers. This response is elicited at very small energy levels, of the order of a few micrometers, nanometers, or even angstroms. It is reproducible every time energy is introduced into the system. It is important to specify here that all forms of energy have the capacity to bring about this phenomenon of reverse transition of biopolymers, including photonic, thermal, chemical, electrical, and electromagnetic energy. However, it should be noted that mechanical energy is five times more effective in this respect than any other form.

Proteins are therefore capable of performing work if stimulated with energy, including mechanical energy. This is the most effective universal mechanism, which involves the folding or elongation of these biopolymers. This universal mechanism underlies most bioenergetic conversion processes.

This means that anatomical structures like reciprocally stretched cranial membranes, the spinal cord dura mater, ligaments, articular capsules, tendons, aponeuroses, and cartilages—in short, all fascial elements found in the human body—are capable at the infinitely minute level (of the order of micrometers, nanometers, or even angstroms) of being induced to retract under the influence of elevated pressure, and subsequently to return to their initial dimensions if the physiological pressure of the surrounding medium is restored.

These scientific discoveries lend concrete support to the osteopathic theory handed down by the masters who have always claimed that osteopathic methods can have profound effects on cellular metabolic processes.

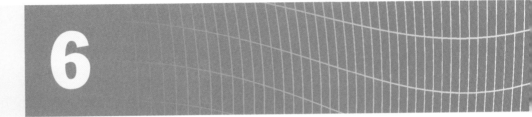

Fascial Mechanics

THE MECHANICAL BEHAVIOR of the fasciae plays an essential role in all bodily functions and in the maintenance of the anatomical integrity of its various parts. In the final analysis, the fascial system functions as a unit, but for a better understanding of the underlying mechanisms, we shall first study them at the local level before analyzing the mechanics of the system as a whole (Fig. 6-1).

Local Mechanics

The local mechanics of the fasciae have many and varied consequences, and these tissues perform vital roles in areas as diverse as suspension and protection, retention, separation, shock absorption, and pressure attenuation.

SUSPENSION AND PROTECTION

Suspension

The fascial elements which play a role in suspending the various structures of the body are the internal ones, for example, the mesentery, the ligaments, and the true fasciae. They guarantee internal cohesion by providing points of attachment which keep each organ in its proper place. The resultant support is firm but, in most cases, not rigid, so that each organ retains some degree of mobility, that is, there is some play in the attachment system. Mobility is not only essential for the ability to respond to the diverse forces to which the human body is regularly subject, but also enters into the general context of the mobility of the body itself – mobility which is essential for the full expression of the body's many different functions and physiological processes.

Fig. 6-1   Fascial Mechanics

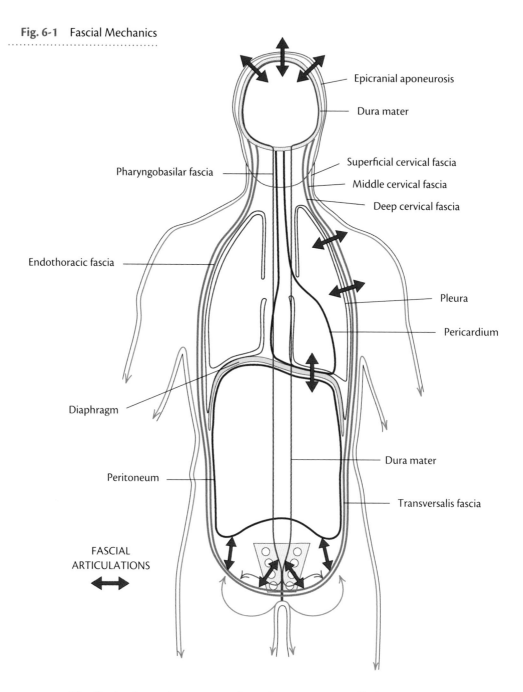

Epicranial aponeurosis

Dura mater

Pharyngobasilar fascia

Superficial cervical fascia

Middle cervical fascia

Deep cervical fascia

Endothoracic fascia

Pleura

Pericardium

Diaphragm

Dura mater

Peritoneum

Transversalis fascia

FASCIAL
ARTICULATIONS

The fascia play an important role in the suspension of other structures, not only in the body cavities, but also in the periphery (Fig. 6-2). Fascial elements such as the aponeuroses and ligaments constitute the support system for all the muscles and joints, whereas the true fasciae support all the vessels and nerves. This all-encompassing peripheral system invests and provides points of attachment for all the vessels, nerves, muscles, and joints, and is itself anchored at fixed points on the bones. Thus, the fascial system plays a central role in maintaining the anatomical integrity of the body as a whole and its component structures.

Fig. 6-2   Fascial Suspension

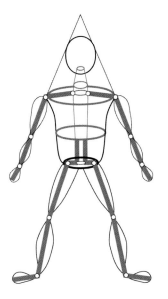

The integrity of the structure of bone tissue depends on the functional state of the tissue itself and, by extension, on the physiological condition of the body as a whole. By itself, a bone is useless—its functionality and its interactions with other skeletal elements depend exclusively on the means of attachment that unite it to neighboring bones.

It appears then that, although the skeleton provides the framework and the anchor points, it is nevertheless completely dependent on soft tissues for maintenance of its cohesion and function. Therefore, there is an inevitable, reciprocal interdependence between the skeleton and the soft tissues—and thereby between structure and function and function and structure.

The role of the fasciae in suspending other structures varies according to the region of the body under consideration. The fasciae have different capacities for stretching in different locations, for example, the skin can stretch ten times more than can a tendon—this reflects the fact that the tendon is composed of type I fibers arranged in parallel, whereas a variety of different types of fiber are present in the skin and the bundles run in all directions. The thickness of collagen fibers is organ-specific, but also changes with age. The elasticity of the fasciae tends to decrease with age. There is thickening, shortening, and calcification of the fibers as a result of all the forces resisted, and the damage inflicted, in earlier years.

The function of suspension shows remarkable adaptability to different situations. Thus, during pregnancy the uterus becomes enormously distended, which necessitates lengthening of all the associated ligaments—without any kind of pain. Not only is the uterus distended, but it pushes into the abdominal cavity, distending the fasciae of the abdominal wall, again without causing any pain. In other, nonphysiological situations in which the uterine ligaments are subjected to stress and tension, they respond by becoming thicker and undergoing calcification; nothing like this happens during pregnancy.

After parturition, the uterus reverts gradually to its normal state, that is, it retracts to recover its original tonus and elasticity. This phenomenon is pre-programmed and may lead one to think that the fasciae have some kind of mechanical 'memory'.

Let us look at the case of obesity, a condition that may be considered pathological. Some people put on an enormous amount of weight, resulting in an accumulation of adipose tissue at all levels. The considerable increase in volume necessitates distension of the fasciae to contain the surplus tissue. However, when the weight is lost again, especially if the process is gradual, the fasciae nearly always regain all their original tonus and elasticity. Is this not an altogether remarkable example of adaptation?

There are other examples. The kidney is contained in a fascial sac which is suspended by various ligaments and the renal artery. If the system of suspension becomes loosened, the organ experiences prolapse and the renal artery becomes stretched. However, the kidney can be successfully restored to its normal position by osteopathic manipulation and, provided that this is done in time, the kidney is soon re-established in its correct position and its supporting structures regain their tonus.

The fasciae demonstrate a remarkable degree of malleability that permits them to adapt constantly to the forces to which they are subject. However, they are also capable of reverting to their original configuration because they are 'pre-programmed' to recognize the body's normal physiological state, as long as they are given some outside assistance within a reasonable time frame.

Protection

In addition to their role in maintenance, the fasciae also underlie a protective mechanism which guarantees the physical and physiological integrity of the body. The mechanism of protection depends on a number of different factors and is based not only on the solidity, but also on the contractility and elasticity of the fasciae.

Maintaining anatomical integrity.

The fasciae, by virtue of their strength, protect the anatomical integrity of the different parts of the body and help the organs preserve their shape. This does not depend on complete rigidity but, on the contrary, is the result of flexibility and adaptability. The exact degree of suppleness varies between different parts of the body.

Thus, the fasciae that invest the kidneys and the liver, or those that maintain the structure of the arteries, although endowed with a measure of elastic potential, have much stronger tonus than the fasciae of the intestines, stomach, veins, and urethra. These are all organs that are subject to variations of shape and pressure, depending on their state of fullness.

Fasciae which must constantly adjust their dimensions to accommodate variations in tension tend to have a particular type of composition, with relatively high densities of reticular and elastic fibers, and a less dense ground substance.

Maintenance of the shape of the muscles is also dependent on the fasciae but, in this case, the fasciae tend to be much denser and stronger. This makes them less prone to deformation so they are more suitable for providing the kind of solid support that muscles need to generate force.

Protecting against changes in tension

The fasciae constitute the first line of defense against significant variations in tension and absorb shocks so as to protect the integrity of the structures that they invest and support. They act just like real shock absorbers which, by virtue of their properties of contractility and elasticity, attenuate the forces to which the body is subject, absorbing and dissipating the energy of severe shocks to preclude damage to the organ with which they are associated.

This protective and buffering activity is most evident in the case of the meninges, the membranous sheets which are designed to preserve the cerebrospinal axis from shocks and sudden variations in pressure that might damage delicate nervous tissue. An additional element is involved in this region to reinforce the shock absorbing activity of the meninges, namely, the cerebrospinal fluid. In the periphery, at particularly sensitive sites such as the kidneys and the ischiorectal fossa, a similar function is provided by adipose tissue which is, in effect, just another, more fluid variety of connective tissue.

It should be recalled that contractility and elasticity are two important factors in the mechanical functioning of the fasciae and that the elasticity of these tissues tends to decrease with age—this phenomenon is, in fact, an important factor in the aging process as a whole. A good example of this is the gradual changes that occur in the skin with aging. When part of the skin is pinched, a fold is formed; this fold will disappear, but it does so more and more slowly with advancing age. The rate of disappearance of the fold provides a measurement of the strength of the covalent cross-links between the fibers, and hence of the overall elasticity of the connective tissue.

The dynamics and the mechanics of a given connective tissue depend on the local concentration of proteoglycans and hyaluronic acid. The rate of proteoglycan synthesis and metabolism can be affected by both intrinsic (heredity, spontaneous mutations) and extrinsic (malnutrition, stress, microbial infections, physical injury) factors.

In response to sustained, abnormal forces, the ground substance can become denser and the collagen fibers may become consolidated to induce a complete change in the structure of the connective tissue, particularly at the points of insertion. If such abnormal forces are sustained over the long term, calcification may ensue. Thus, certain attachments to ligaments and fasciae become progressively more calcified when exposed to severe and persistent tension. This phenomenon occurs especially frequently in and around the calcaneus, the elbow, the shoulder, and the vertebral column, to just mention a few cases which are often encountered in clinical practice.

To counter the effects of constant irritation, inflammation, and other serious, repeated types of insult, the connective tissue has developed a defensive mechanism based on its transformation into bone tissue. This represents an extraordinary system of adaptation and compensation, all the more remarkable in that the effects are completely reversible. This topic will be discussed in more detail later.

RETENTION AND SEPARATION

> "The fasciae unite and separate everything, separate and unite everything"
>
> —L. Issartel

Retention

There is not a single part of the body that is not invested by some kind of fascial element. The study of anatomy demonstrates that the human body is constituted of large envelopes that enclose more or less extensive regions. Within these major compartments, there are additional fasciae to enclose ever finer sub-structures without, however, creating any kind of discontinuity. For example, in the thigh, a single, large cylindrical sheath invests all the muscles of that region as a unit. However, this large cylinder is sub-divided into multiple compartments by intermuscular septa, which separate different groups of muscles with different functions. Inside each of these sub-compartments, groups of muscles are invested by another kind of sheath of fascial tissue which demarcates individual muscles. Inside each muscle, yet another fascial sheet surrounds each bundle of muscle fibers which, in turn, are compartmentalized by yet another level of membrane enclosing the individual myofibrils.

The abdominal cavity is lined by a large membranous sac that contains all the viscera, isolating them from neighboring structures and thus maintaining a certain cohesion as well as insuring constant pressure. This structure, the peritoneum, is, however, also subdivided into mesenteriesa and ligaments that constitute the structural envelopes of the various organs.

The function of the fasciae is thus to maintain the anatomical structure of the soft tissues. The fasciae are at one and the same time a structural component, support unit, and framework. Any weakness of the fasciae may lead to herniation of the internal organs and other structures. Such herniation may lead to rupture and impairment of physiological function.

The organs could not fulfill their functions in the absence of the fasciae. Hollow organs would be massively distended, and their function would be compromised beyond recovery, given the fact that the epithelia of all organs are anchored in basement membranes and this configuration is essential for normal tissue turnover. An artery devoid of fasciae would be flaccid and easily occluded by the slightest compression—the circulatory system would be completely nonfunctional. Any of the fluid-filled organs, deprived of its fascial framework, would be unable to maintain its shape and would similarly be completely nonfunctional.

Without fascial support, muscles would be unable to generate any force from contraction. As has been pointed out, the fasciae have a more or less inelastic, rigid structure. A muscle, when contracting, requires points of support to have any effect. These points of support are created by bridges which anchor them to the bones, but these alone would be insufficient (especially when contraction includes the displacement of one segment with respect to another) if the muscles were not also supported by fasciae. The fasciae not only provide points of attachment for the muscles, but also points of support, which permit the muscles to realize their full power.

The retention function of the fasciae also serves to protect organs and muscles against shocks and sudden variations in pressure by absorbing some of the energy. Without this capacity for retention, these structures would soon suffer from tears and other injuries.

The fascial retention function is also important in the channeling of physiological forces: without the fasciae, movement would be impossible to produce, control, or coordinate.

Separation

All anatomic structures are linked by fasciae, but these same elements are also a means for separating structures without any loss of cohesion.

Separation is brought about by compartmentalization and the creation of planes of cleavage.

Cleavage

Planes of cleavage serve to avoid rigidity and to retain the mobility that is a fundamental requirement for even the tiniest structures of the body. They also help endow any given organ or structure with some degree of independence from its neighbors. Every part of the body, while remaining in intimate contact with its neighbors, is also separated from them by planes of cleavage. These consist of areas of areolar connective tissue that fill the spaces between organs and also, as previously noted, link structures together.

There are two main points of interest regarding planes of cleavage:

- They help organs, entire muscles, and individual bundles of muscle fibers slide over one other. This allows for changes in shape and tension, and makes coordinated movement possible.
- They represent crossing-over points where deep palpation is possible.

When, in the course of tests and treatments, we want to examine deep-seated zones, we have to traverse the barrier represented by the muscles. When we attempt to penetrate such a layer of muscle tissue, we are frustrated by resistance due to the tension of the muscle, that is, its reflex contraction. In other words, there is a thick, dense structure between our hand and the area of interest—this makes palpation difficult or completely impossible.

Planes of cleavage make it possible to bypass this barrier. Thus, if one wants to palpate the piriformis muscle or the sacrospinal ligament, one must make use of the cleavage plane between the gluteus maximus and the gluteus medius muscles. If one wants to palpate the sciatic nerve at the posterior face of the thigh, the only possible approach is the cleavage plane between the adductor and hamstring muscles. Likewise, in order to palpate a kidney, the only effective approach is via the meeting point between the external edge of the rectus muscle and the oblique muscle of the abdomen.

If one wants to palpate a common anterior vertebral ligament, the only possible approach is via the linea alba. However, it should be remembered that this point of cleavage is subject to variation; for example, during pregnancy, displacement of the linea alba is an important factor in the ability of the abdomen to undergo the massive distension which is necessary. But unfortunately, sometimes, imperfect postpartum re-joining results in separation of the different constituent layers of the linea alba so that the intestinal loops can easily be felt through it.

Finally, being familiar with the pattern of cleavage planes in the abdominal cavity makes it possible for the surgeon to make smaller incisions and still be able to clearly separate the various organs from one other.

Compartmentalization

Repeated splitting and division of the fascial sheets generates a complex network of more or less isolated compartments. This makes it possible to maintain different pressures in different places, and also helps block the spread of infections or inflammatory mediators from one part of an organ to another.

This compartmentalization protects organs from the spread of abscesses in surrounding tissue. However, as we have seen, there is also segmentation within the organs: the most typical example is the separate lobes comprising the liver and lung. The aim of this additional compartmentalization is to protect the vital organs and to ensure that their functions continue to be performed even when part of the organ has been damaged. Thus, for example, a liver can still perform its physiological role as long as at least 30% of the original functional tissue is operational.

ABSORPTION OF SHOCKS

When the body is subject to any kind of violent trauma at the surface, a shock wave is generated which propagates towards the interior. Such shock waves can conduct and deliver huge amounts of energy to the deep tissues, thereby causing serious damage to many different internal structures and organs if the intensity of the original shock is strong enough.

The role of connective tissue is to absorb that shock wave and to dissipate it in different directions so as to attenuate it and protect the physical integrity of the body. If the intensity of the shock exceeds a certain threshold, the connective tissue can no longer absorb enough of the energy and injury will result, possibly fatal; the most common fatal injuries are rupture of the spleen or the liver, and fracture of the kidney.

By virtue of the orientation of the fascial fibers, connective tissue acts as a buffer and disperses the energy in different directions so as to attenuate the intensity of the shock wave and absorb its energy.

In certain situations, however, the energy cannot be fully absorbed and dissipated. Either the shock was too violent or it struck an area which was already subject to abnormal tension. What can occur in this case is the formation of what Elmer Green has called an "energy cyst," that is, the concentration of a significant amount of energy within the connective tissue, energy that sooner or later will have deleterious effects. Such a cyst of energy manifests by obstructing the normal conduction of electricity through the tissues of the body. It acts like an irritant, which can contribute to the development of an area which is a propitious focus for the kind of phenomena conventionally associated with irritation. This leads to an increase in entropy and loss of function in the surrounding tissues. A cyst of energy can result from trauma, invasion by a pathogen, physiological dysfunction, or even emotional stress.

It seems strange that soft tissue can, by itself, accumulate an amount of energy that remains imprisoned within it. We have seen that the role of the ground substance is partly that of a shock absorber, and that, in order to accomplish this task, it exploits a number of different mechanisms to restore its normal physiological status after a compromising event. In certain situations these mechanisms are insufficient and the ground substance can no longer fully resolve the stress. It then retains the memory of the stress in an autonomous manner, independent of any higher control mechanism. To be sure, the higher control system may intervene in order to enhance the possibility of discharging the energy, and thereby avoid sequelae, but it cannot obliterate the stress

This is demonstrated by Frankstein's experiment, as noted in Korr. A cat, when injected in the paw with oil of turpentine, will immediately place its paw in the position of triple withdrawal. With time, the cat recovers normal use of its paw. When, several months later, the cat is decerebrated, the injured paw immediately resumes the triple withdrawal position. Interruption of the higher regulatory processes has brought the original trauma back out again in the present. One speaks here of cellular or peripheral memory, more specifically of "ground substance memory."

When the buffering capacity of connective tissue is overwhelmed, that is, when a traumatic insult or any other kind of injury has surpassed a certain intensity, local stress sets in. Usually it develops, sometimes over a period of years, without any symptoms; but ultimately, in most cases, some kind of disease state will result. This occurs by means of an autonomous local mechanism but, through the intermediary of the nervous system, such a phenomenon can quickly spread to a much broader area. This involves the mechanism of spinal segment facilitation.

In a facilitated spinal segment, resistance to the conduction of electrical impulses is reduced. The segment is highly irritable, and any additional stimulus—even a very weak one—will bring about a strong response, the magnitude of which is out of all proportion to the intensity of the additional stimulus.

The segment where facilitation has occurred will induce modifications in the tonus of the muscle associated with it, which will be associated with a concomitant reduction in the mobility of the segment as well as a palpable change in tissue structure. It may be recalled that this change can be induced directly—bypassing the reflex arc—through modification of the composition of the ground substance. Such impaired ground substance function will have repercussions at the surface of the skin through the intermediary of the "Heine cylinders" (see chapter 3, page 130).

Sympathetic stimulation, in turn, leads to a change in the texture of the skin as well as to changes in the activity of the sweat glands. Eventually, the problem will spread distally to organs that depend on the metameric territory, which will also become dysfunctional in the absence of outside intervention. A facilitated segment, unfortunately, has a tendency to self-perpetuate and spread.

ABSORPTION OF PRESSURE

The body is subject at all times to tensions, pulling forces, shocks, and stresses of many different kinds. It is unlikely that the human being would be viable—in any case, its functions would be greatly impaired—if there were no defensive barrier capable of absorbing potentially damaging forces.

The shock absorbing role is in great part mediated by the fasciae and is dependent on the biochemical composition of this special kind of tissue, especially on its elastic components, on its special anatomical structure, and on the presence of the adipose tissue cushions which are part of it.

Biochemical composition

We have seen in the preceding chapters how the buffering capacity of connective tissue derives from the composition of the ground substance, especially its proteoglycan content. It should be recalled that the proteoglycans modify the viscoelastic properties of tissues, the properties which are most important in determining how they respond to changes in pressure.

The ratio of ground substance to fibers depends on the forces to which a tissue is subject. Thus, in a ligament which is subject to strong forces but always in the same direction, the ground substance will be relatively sparse, while the fibers will be very abundant and aligned in parallel bundles along the axis of the predominant force.

The result of the buffering activity of the fasciae is to attenuate the intensity of any potentially damaging force and to absorb some of the energy, whatever the nature of the original insult. If stress persists, the fasciae will modify their structure in response to it. Thus, wherever any tension is applied in a sustained manner, the collagen fibers increase in number and align themselves in the direction of the force. This can eventually give rise to fibrosis.

Hurschler et al., in studies of pathological fasciae, particularly in patients with anterior tibial compartment syndrome, did not find any differences in the absolute amount of collagen present; they did, however, observe an increase in the thickness of the fibers as well as increased rigidity.

There is, in the case of pathological fasciae, a decrease in the extent to which the fibers are cross-linked. In some patients, the fibers appear to be thickened; in others, they appear both thickened and adhesions to muscles were detected; and in a third group, the fibers appeared histologically normal. This makes us think that each subject responds in a different manner to the same kind of pathology, probably according to their overall "state of health." When dealing with an individual, one must therefore integrate the disease in a holistic context. This is what Korr is referring to when he says "there are no illnesses, but only ill people."

Page notes that connective tissue forms the membranes across which the osmotic processes of nutrition and elimination occur. Abnormal pressures and tensions will therefore also have an impact on the osmotic exchanges between different fluid compartments.

The equilibrium between the circulating blood and the tissue fluids must be maintained so that the physiological balance of the body can find its full expression. Any membrane tension can disturb the hemodynamic processes of the body, with the result that the efficiency of tissue drainage will be reduced and metabolites will begin to accumulate. This will inevitably lead to progressive local dysfunction. Yahia et al. prepared specimens from pathological lumbar fasciae and observed marked thickening with re-orientation of all the fibers in the same direction.

Elastic components

A fascia is not a totally rigid structure. Wherever it is observed, it always has some degree of elasticity which allows it to attenuate pressure and increases its breaking point. In the course of violent exertion, the muscles are supported and reinforced by elastic connective tissue. Without some elasticity in the system, the muscles would soon reach their breaking point and irreparable damage would result. In practice, rupture is rare, evidence of the powerful viscoelastic and contractile potential of the fascial system.

Yahia et al. studied the effect of stretching forces on specimens of fascial tissue. They found that the more the fasciae were stretched, the more rigid they became; thus, in order to obtain the same given deformation in a shorter period of time, a greater load had to be used. Furthermore, if the fasciae were submitted to a constant load, the extent of deformation steadily decreased over time.

Adipose tissue

In addition to its roles in fat storage and thermal insulation, adipose tissue also acts as a shock absorber. The importance of this kind of tissue in that function varies among different parts of the body.

In the skin, adipose tissue acts as a cushion which attenuates the intensity of shocks, although its efficacy in this respect depends on its thickness, which varies from region to region. Thus, a blow on the arm, where there is a relatively thick layer of adipose tissue, is much less painful than a blow on the tibial face of the calf, where there is practically none.

In the abdomen, in addition to filling the spaces between the various organs, internal cushions of adipose tissue significantly attenuate the pressures that are normally generated inside the abdominal cavity. This protects all the organs so that they can continue functioning normally.

Around the kidney, there is a particularly thick layer of adipose tissue. In addition to keeping the kidney in place (prolapse of the kidney is common during rapid weight loss when fat around the kidney is eliminated too quickly), this adipose pad protects the organ from physical trauma which, if violent enough, could cause its rupture.

There are considerable amounts of adipose tissue associated with the perineum, which, in view of its location, role, and anatomical structure, warrants special attention. It perfectly illustrates a number of different key properties of the fasciae. As a brief reminder, the perineum is composed of three superimposed layers of fasciae: the superficial perineal fascia, the middle fascia of the anterior perineum, and the deep perineal fascia that corresponds to the sheet of tissue that seals the abdominal cavity. These fascial envelopes invest a variety of different muscles that reinforce and underlie them.

This construction would be perfect if it did not include gaps in the anteroposterior direction where the special structures of the true pelvis are located, that is, the rectum, the bladder, and, in females, the vagina. The vagina is a major introversion in which both the cervix of the uterus and the neck of the bladder are situated.

The central part of the perineum is filled, in the anteroposterior direction, by the structures of the true pelvis, all of which are more or less concave in shape. The perineum is attached to these structures and is supported by them. Laterally, there is a pair of longitudinal structures, the ischioanal fossae, which are also filled with adipose tissue.

The perineum represents the most steeply inclined part of the thoracoabdominal cavity and it supports an entire 'fluid' column which contains not only the organs of the actual perineum, but also those of the abdomen and thorax. This represents a considerable weight which, since the perineum is not hermetically sealed, would predispose the perineal organs to prolapse if it all had to be borne in the vertical plane. In fact, such prolapse is actually (and fortunately) a rare event.

To avoid prolapse and to support the overlying visceral column, as well as to make efficient sphincter function possible and absorb the pressures generated locally, the perineum is endowed with several properties and features which serve to protect it:

- elasticity and solidity
- a special anatomical architecture
- an adipose cushion
- additional shock absorbers
- coordinated movement

Elasticity and solidity

In order to support the organs, the perineal fasciae must combine two essential, but apparently mutually exclusive properties, namely, elasticity and solidity:

- solidity to support the enormous pressures that can arise, especially when coughing or in the course of violent exertion
- elasticity in order to absorb the high pressures which are constantly being generated, and also to permit free movement of the sphincters

If either of these qualities is compromised, the function of the perineal organs will be affected. There is a danger of dysfunction of the bladder and the uterus, and, sooner or later, these same organs may experience prolapse.

Special anatomical architecture

It was pointed out that the perineal organs have a roughly concave form in the anteroposterior and sagittal directions. This permits distribution of the pressures from the overlying region in all directions, rather than exclusively vertically. Kamina notes that the "internal static pressures are all the better insofar as the physiological orientation of the genitalia is conserved or accentuated and the supporting elements are solid."

On exertion, because of the overall configuration of the pelvis, intra-abdominal pressure is mainly directed towards the back, that is, towards the very strong anococcygeal region. There is a posterior transfer of pressure from the viscera and, in particular, the uterus, the cervix of which is supported by the posterior perineum.

Furthermore, the levator ani muscles contract to oppose the force generated as a result of the pressure. They lift the tendinous center of the perineum that pushes the posterior vaginal wall in an anterior direction, thus inclining the vagina at an angle to the posterior cul-de-sac, the so-called 'vaginal angle.'

Evidently, when it comes to anatomical architecture, one has to keep in mind the inclination of the pelvis, and the existence of lumbar lordosis and abdominal tonus. Any increase in lumbar lordosis or loss of abdominal tonus will tend to induce anteversion of the pelvis. If this occurs, the resultant forces on the perineum will tend to be focused at the vulval cleft and excessive pressure will be exerted on the bladder and uterus. Weakening of the perineum will very soon lead to prolapse of the neck of the bladder or of the uterine cervix.

Adipose cushion

The adipose tissue in the ischioanal fossae exists not only to fill an empty space and protect the local vessels and nerves, but also to absorb pressure. It acts as an elastic buffer that both attenuates and absorbs pressure.

Additional shock absorbers

The perineal cavity is closed posterolaterally by the piriformis muscle that is invested by fasciae derived from the deep perineal fascia. The piriformis muscle, as well as hermetically sealing the pelvic girdle in the back, constitutes an additional shock absorbing element in the true pelvis.

The pelvis has two lateral openings, the obturator foramina. What purpose do these serve? Apart from providing an insertion point for the two obturator muscles, they are filled with the obturator membrane, an elastic sheet that vibrates in response to pressure on the true pelvis, rather like the gills of a fish. These structures therefore constitute an additional force-modulating system.

Coordinated movement

It should not be forgotten that the true pelvis lies below a significant visceral mass in the abdomen, and that this abdominal mass is confined at the top by the piston-action diaphragm, which is constantly moving up and down. Part of the resultant pressure on the visceral column is transmitted down towards the organs of the pelvis. The soft tissues of the perineum, by virtue of their elasticity, absorb and compensate for this constant movement and thereby preclude damage to internal structures.

There is then some degree of coordination with the diaphragm in the form of a slight downward movement during inhalation. This may be demonstrated by breathing at the same time as the perineum is being contracted: you will see that breathing immediately becomes more difficult and you will be able to feel the increase in pressure. Overall, thanks to the solidity, plasticity, and viscoelastic properties of the fasciae, the pressure transmitted by the thoracoabdominal column is not all exerted vertically, but is distributed to and supported by all the various components of the pelvic girdle:

- Below and behind, at the level of the central fibrous ring of the perineum, is the most acutely inclined cavity, where all of the fasciae and most of the perineal muscles converge. It serves as the thread which closes the bag and may be considered the most solid point.
- Laterally there is a primary shock absorber in the form of a pad of adipose tissue. Still more laterally, there are the obturator membranes in front and the piriformis muscles further back.
- Finally, in front, some of the force is absorbed by the anterior peritoneum and the symphysis.

Anatomical design

The fasciae, anchored to the skeleton, are not a simple tube composed of perfectly parallel vertical bands. The architecture of the fasciae consists of several superimposed, interdependent layers, arranged in vertical, horizontal, and oblique configurations to enhance the tissue's solidity and potentiate its capacity to resist any force to which it is exposed.

Debnar et al. analyzed specimens of thoracolumbar fascial tissue and demonstrated that they are composed of numerous laminae of collagen fibers, each arranged at a different angle with respect to the others. Gerlach and Lierse studied the fasciae of the lower limbs and found the following (Fig. 6-3):

Fig. 6-3   Fasciae of the Lower Limb (after Gerlach)

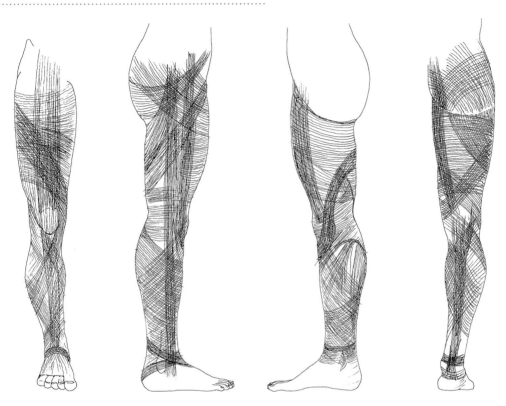

▶ ANTERIOR FASCIAE HAVE:

- horizontally oriented fibers, some of which are attached to the iliotibial tract, with others disappearing posteriorly
- vertically disposed fibers in the upper part of the thigh; these fibers are interwoven with the horizontal fibers
- obliquely disposed fibers, lower down and on the inside, with their lower ends continuing into the interior of the tibia. These fibers are thinner than the vertical ones, except at the level of the hip, where they are stronger

▶ POSTERIOR FASCIAE HAVE:

- strong, vertically disposed fibers
- horizontally disposed fibers, especially dense below the gluteus maximus muscle and in the lower part of the thigh, where they terminate in the popliteal fossa

The lowest fibers are archiform, at first obliquely disposed below and inside, and then vertical; they continue via the aponeurosis of the posterior tibial muscle.

▶ INTERNAL FASCIAE HAVE:

- both vertically and obliquely disposed fibers, the latter originating from the fascia lata
- an anterior group of obliquely disposed fibers below and in front, and a posterior group of similarly disposed fibers below and behind. The anterior fibers merge with the patellar retinaculum, and the lateral fibers with the medial collateral ligament. The internal lateral part consists of very dense, extremely strong fibers which are easy to palpate.

▶ EXTERNAL FASCIAE HAVE:

- very powerful, vertically disposed fibers which form the iliotibial tract. This tract is linked to the femur by the external interosseous membrane.

The inferior fasciae form part of the patellar retinaculum and of the external lateral ligament. The fibers of the thigh continue into the leg and the foot where they show the same basic structural pattern.

The fasciae of the lower limbs and, in fact, the fasciae in general, have an overall spiral configuration which permits them to act like a 'floor cloth' which 'soaks up' fluid, as was previously discussed. Furthermore, this design increases their ability to resist force and maintain the body's normal anatomical structure.

General Mechanics

NERVOUS CONDUCTION OF PAIN

Pain impulses from the periphery are conducted to the dorsal horn of the spinal cord. From there, the signal is routed via tracts inside the spinal cord to specific higher central nervous system centers which process the information and then send back an appropriate response. This outline is highly simplified, and the real situation is far more complex: there is actually a whole network of peripheral receptors which send signals along anatomically characterized pathways, but it seems that conduction channels are not as simple as one might think, and that there are important circuits which we do not understand at all.

Not all the information arriving at the dorsal horn of the spinal cord induces a response because we are in a state of constant nervous stimulation. For a reaction, it is necessary that there be a series of different, corroborative signals; on the basis of this observation, Melzach and Wall developed the gate theory.

In the dorsal horn of the spinal cord there is a regulatory mechanism to increase or decrease the rate at which nervous impulses are transmitted. This mechanism depends on the activity of A-beta and A-delta nerve fibers, as well as signals coming down from the brain. When the quantity of information passing through the gate exceeds a certain threshold, the regions of the brain responsible for pain sensation become activated.

A flow of impulses arrive at the tract cells of the dorsal horn and, up to a certain threshold of tolerance, these cells exert an inhibitory activity and the gate remains closed. When the accumulation of signals exceeds the threshold, the inhibition is lifted, the gate opens, and pain is felt.

However, the idea of a purely spinal mechanism poses certain problems. The gate theory is based on presynaptic control but it is known that there are also postsynaptic inhibitory mechanisms. This is evidence of a back-up mechanism, but also indicates that lesional triggering occurs, and certainly in the periphery before intervention of the reflex arc. Therefore, it would appear that not all the information passes through the higher centers, but that some is treated by the 'peripheral brain.' Experiments have shown that rats are still able to learn to find their way through a maze in search of food even after decerebration. The spinal cord has its own memory, and can both take decisions and solve problems.

It is important to note that this peripheral brain function is also found in the fasciae. The fasciae are channels for the conduction of superficial sensory stimuli which follows a path other than that involving the spinal cord. As far back as the early nineteenth century, Bichat called this phenomenon 'intermembrane sympathy.' For example, if the thigh is scratched, irritation can be felt at some remote point, like on the back.

This peripheral conduction of sensitivity is perfectly illustrated by the phenomenon of causalgia. This condition can induce pain so acute that some victims are driven to commit suicide. Moreover, in some of the most refractory cases, while radicotomy, sympathectomy, cordotomy, or sectioning of the spinal cord may give temporary remission, the pain can return to the same degree. Where does it come from and where does it pass through? Definitely not the nervous system of the spinal cord, because that has been eliminated.

It seems that there exists an autonomous sensory network which constitutes the primary peripheral organization and which functions in an entirely independent manner. Lightly touching a sensitive area can trigger acute pain, and sometimes the pain will manifest without any obvious stimulus at all. Pain can spread in an unpredictable way to distant parts of the body which have no relationship with the initial focus of pain.

Often, pain persists long after the triggering stimulus has disappeared. This phenomenon escapes any kind of logical explanation if only a specific, rigid, and direct sensory system is considered. Thus, normally, a half-full bladder is not felt and does not induce the desire to urinate. Fullness induces the urination response by stimulating mechanoreceptors. However, patients with cystitis feel the need to urinate even when the bladder is far from full.

The uterus is doubly innervated. Its body is innervated by a group of fibers from the thoracolumbar region and is only painful in the event of massive dilatation, serious infection, during delivery, and, in certain women, at the time of menstruation. Certainly, in the last case, the fasciae are in a state of maximum summation and the simple fact of menstrual congestion suffices to trigger the pain.

The cervix is innervated by the hypogastric plexus and is a focus of intense pain if it is dilated by even a few centimeters. Not only do different tissues react differently to stimuli but, within even the same organ, the reactions to the same kind of stimulus can be completely different.

It seems ever more evident that the fasciae are not only the focus of sensitivity, but that they are also capable of independently processing information. Pischinger attributes this capacity to a fundamental system. It is guaranteed by the homeostatic mechanisms of the system, that is, correction with a minimum loss of energy, mistakes resulting from the intrusion of perturbing factors.

These perturbing factors usually act in a unilateral fashion, only compromising mobility and function in the affected segment. Even before the appearance of frank, clinical symptoms, the disturbance is already well-established and already entails the expenditure of more energy to maintain normal functionality. Then, by a segmental reflex channel, the involvement spreads more deeply, perhaps even to the viscera. Finally, a chronic condition is established and the entire side of the body may become involved and dysfunctional.

Yahia et al., studying the thoracolumbar fascia, discovered the presence of corpuscles of Ruffini and Paccini. Ruffini's corpuscles are characterized by a simple axon with very dense dendritic network containing collagen fibers. Mechanoreceptors are mainly concentrated around blood vessels and in areolar connective tissue with bundles of dense collagen fibers.

Nervous conduction in the fasciae seems to be part of the sympathetic system, which is important not only in the mechanics but also in the biochemistry of the tissues. To a lesser extent, the parasympathetic system is also involved. The sympathetic system controls the circulation and metabolic activity and has an enormous influence on pH and on the elimination of waste products.

If the fasciae have their own innervation, it means that they are not rigid but capable of some level of motion. This has been investigated by Yahia et al., who studied explanted specimens of fascial tissue. They showed that stretching induced spontaneous contraction, that is, an increase in the viscoelasticity of the tissue in response to the insult.

Boabighi et al. showed that collagen fibers contain regular undulations, the shape of which is comparable to the waves formed at the surface of moving fluids. The mean amplitude of these undulations was 6 micrometers, and their mean wave length was 60 micrometers (Table 6-1).

Therefore, the fasciae should be considered as structures which are capable of some degree of autonomous motion. The source of this motion should be sought in the embryo. Embryological development is nothing more than a state of perpetual motion which, in the end, results in the construction of a human being.

Remember, as discussed at length in Chapter 1, that at the very beginning of life, there are three different but intimately associated layers of tissue, namely, the ectoderm, the mesoderm, and the endoderm. These three layers migrate to form the skeleton, the cavities, and the organs. These migrations occur simultaneously. Each layer migrates in a coordinated way and interacts and interpenetrates its neighbors. A 'memory' of this perpetual motion will persist, and this memory can be detected in the cranium, the viscera, and the fasciae. Its amplitude is somewhere between eight and fourteen periods per minute, with a certain degree of variation between different parts of the body. This perpetual motion facilitates cellular exchange processes and acts as a pump to drive fluids around the body.

It would seem that this motion is maintained by the sympathetic nervous system, and that any change in its rhythm—an increase, decrease, or its disappearance—represents an important diagnostic aid, as will be discussed in detail later on.

Table 6-1 Histological Properties of the Fasciae

STRUCTURE	Fiber Diameter (micrometers)	Amplitude (micrometers)	Wavelength (micrometers)
Brachial aponeurosis	130	8.5	30
Antebrachial aponeurosis	155	8.5	30
Extensor retinaculum	200	1.5	70
Flexor retinaculum	200	1.5	70
Upper aponeurosis of the external oblique m.	155	8.5	30
Lower aponeurosis of the external oblique m.	170	5.7	85
Anterior fascia lata	150	8.5	30
Iliotibial tract	155	4.5	75
Ankle extensor retinaculum	285	1.5	80

MORPHOLOGICAL CHARACTERISTICS

Connective tissue is rich in collagen fibers assembled into dense, almost parallel bundles, the orientation of which follows the direction in which mechanical forces tend to be imposed. The difference in intensity between mechanical forces leads us to observe, in a general way:

- In the upper limb, the anterolateral fasciae tend to be thicker and stronger than the posteromedial ones.
- The same kind of tendency is observed in the lower limb, apart from within the leg, where the anteromedial fascia covering the tibia is the thickest of all.
- In the palms of the hands and soles of the feet, the fasciae are extremely thick and strong.
- In the neck and trunk, as a rule the posterior fasciae are stronger than the anterior fasciae.

This difference in various parts of the body can be explained by their biomechanical characteristics. The thickest, strongest fasciae either have to work harder or have a tough retention function to perform. They are the most important in maintaining posture and form. As previously noted, it is the intensity of the force to which they are subject which determines the characteristics of different fasciae, so the differences observed appear to be entirely logical. Boabighi et al. have studied the biomechanical properties of various fasciae (*Table 6-2*).

Table 6-2 Biomechanical Properties of Certain Fascial Elements

STRUCTURE	Lengthening (%)	Strain (N/mm2)	Deformation [Young's module] (N/mm2)
Brachial aponeurosis	88	1.7	2
Bicipital aponeurosis	42	2.9	12
Antebrachial aponeurosis	43	1.2	3
Extensor retinaculum	55	1.0	3
Flexor retinaculum	76	1.3	2
Palmar aponeurosis	47	2.4	7
Digital fascia	53	2.6	13
Aponeurosis of the external oblique m.	100	1.2	3
Lower aponeurosis of the internal oblique m.	62	2.5	18
Fascia lata	48	0.6	2
Iliotibial tract	35	3.8	19
Ankle extensor retinaculum	65	1.1	3

Analysis of these results shows that the breaking strength of one group of fasciae is as high as Young's module. This group includes the bicipital aponeurosis, the palmar and digital fasciae, the iliotibial tract, and the inferior aponeurosis of the external oblique muscle. Moreover, this same group has mean values which are lower for stretching and corresponds to those fascial elements which were classified above as among the thickest and strongest.

Morphological analysis reveals:

- that the lower limbs have a natural tendency towards external rotation
- that the upper limbs have a natural tendency towards internal rotation

In Chapter 7 on fascial tests, it will be seen that this general tendency can sometimes be distorted.

Another remarkable particularity concerns the alignment of the extremities with respect to the trunk. While the lower limbs are in series with the trunk and the pelvis, the upper limbs seem to be connected in parallel to the thorax, like grafts that have been stuck on to the body. The practical relevance of this observation will be dealt with later.

MAINTAINING POSTURE

Although the muscular system is central in the maintenance and correction of posture, the muscles cannot achieve this task without the intimate participation of the fasciae. As previously noted, no muscle can be functional without the fascial system. Moreover, in some instances, the fasciae completely take over from muscles in the maintenance of posture.

With respect to this role, certain fasciae are more active than others. Cathie (1974) mentions the following fasciae: the gluteal, cervical, and lumbosacral fasciae, and the iliotibial tract. He observed clearly visible bands on these fascial elements, which confirms that the harder a fascial element has to work, the more it will consolidate its collagen network. This is why the fasciae are the first structures to react to injury.

Recent histological results support the hypothesis that the thoracolumbar fascia may play a sensory role in the vertebral column mechanism. On anterior flexion of the trunk, no additional electrical activity is observed in the posterior muscles. Their action is supplanted by the vertebral ligaments.

If the muscles are the motors of posture, it would seem that they intervene in a more obvious way in the dynamic situation. Insofar as the static situation is concerned, the fasciae seem to be more important for maintaining position—the virtue of which is that it saves energy.

As a general rule, it is the external fasciae that are involved in maintaining posture, while the internal fasciae tend to be more important in support functions. In addition, their anatomy and architecture show that they are ideally suited for maintaining posture.

FASCIAL CHAINS

General remarks

Anatomical analysis of the fasciae clearly shows us that the system is continuous from the cranium to the feet. As previously noted, there are both internal and external fascial chains, each communicating with the other. There is never any kind of interruption in the fascial system; each gives into the next in a completely harmonious sequence. They simply form a series of transfer points on the bones to enhance their cohesion and improve their efficacy. Depending on the orientation of the fascial fibers, these chains may be vertical or oblique (Fig. 6-4).

Vleeming et al., in work on the thoracolumbar fascia, showed that its superficial lamina was continuous with the aponeurosis of the gluteus maximus. At the level of the sacrum, some of the fibers continue directly on the same side, while others cross over to form a transfer point (sometimes called a relay point) on the posterior superior iliac process and the iliac crest, where they meet with fibers from the aponeurosis of the latissimus dorsi muscle.

The superficial layer joins with the deep layer at the level of the sacrum and continues into the sacrotuberous ligament.

Fig. 6-4   Fascial Chains

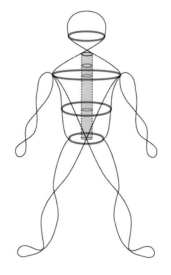

Traction at a given point on the superficial thoracolumbar fascia induces displacement of the fascia to a greater or lesser extent in the direction of the force; this displacement can be contralateral (due to the obliquely disposed fibers). Traction on the biceps femoris and its fascia induces displacement of the deep layer by the sacrotuberous ligament as far as the lower lumbar vertebrae; again, contralateral displacement can occur.

The lumbar fascia can be moved by various muscles, including the latissimus dorsi, hamstrings, abdominal oblique, and the gluteus maximus. The contralateral gluteus maximus and latissimus dorsi muscles create a perpendicular force at the sacroiliac joint. The thoracolumbar fascia transmits forces between the vertebral column, the pelvis, and the lower limb.

This fascial continuity is confirmed by the work of Gerlach and Lierse, who studied the fasciae of the thigh. This begins at the top at the inguinal ligament, iliac crest, sacrum, and coccyx. Its lower part contributes to the ligaments of the knee and continues down into the fasciae of the leg. Moreover, it is connected to the perineum via the intermuscular septa. A lamina of connective tissue emanating from the fascia lata forms the internal and external intermuscular septa. This fixes the fascia lata and the iliotibial tract to the femur, thereby creating a solid unit consisting of bone, fascia, and tendon.

Role of the chains

The role of the chains can be analyzed in terms of three main functions:

- transmission
- coordination and harmonization

• damping

Transmission

For the purpose of simplification, the fasciae can be considered as ropes which transmit forces through the body. Of course, the motor driving this system is muscular contraction, but this only functions when associated with the fasciae.

In order to transmit their energy in an efficient and coordinated fashion, these ropes must be anchored at certain points. These anchor points are usually provided at joints, which act as pulleys for the ropes (*Fig.* 6-5).

Fig. 6-5 Fascial Pulley and Chain systems

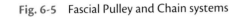

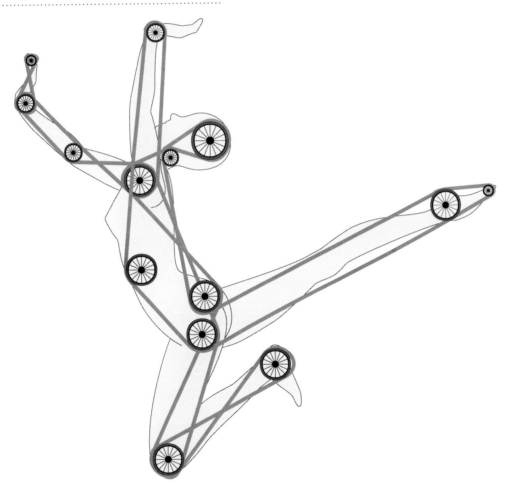

Coordination and harmonization

For any movement to be effective, the energy which produces it must be appropriately channeled. In the case of the body, the muscles also need to be effectively coordinated so that the motor forces can be made to act in concert.

Harmonization and coordination take place at the level of the fasciae. Thus, when executing a complex set of movements like those involved in walking, a whole series of mechanisms which involve the entire body are brought into play.

The first requirement is that the erect position be maintained. This entails permanent, ongoing readjustment of the vertical position with respect to a base, that is, the feet, which represent a relatively limited area of support. The erect position must be maintained with minimum expenditure of energy, which is largely achieved by exploitation of the fascial rope and pulley system.

When it comes to actually walking, a whole set of complex movements must be coordinated in order that progress is made in the desired direction. In other words, one or more fascial chains must be brought into play in order to accomplish an accurate, effective movement. The simple act of walking necessarily entails a whole series of compensatory movements, for example, balancing with the upper limbs, inclination of the trunk, and so on.

It is obvious that if there were no harmonization among all these different movements, even a function as routine as walking would become overly complicated, if not impossible. Of course, a whole array of systems is involved in this harmonization, including the muscles, nerves, and centers of balance. However, it would be impossible without the fasciae.

Every movement that we execute is actually the sum of many different component movements, including flexions, extensions, and rotations. In everyday life, every movement is usually a combination of a number of parameters: the architecture of the fascial fibers with their different arrangements (vertical, oblique, or transverse) seems to be ideally suited to harmonize these combinations of factors so as to render the overall movement functional.

Dampening

The fascial chains transmit the movements of everyday life but are also involved in coping with violent exertion and trauma. In the case of violent exertion, the body as a whole participates to distribute the effects over as extensive an area as possible so that the breaking point of no one part is exceeded. The muscles are there to provide the energy necessary for the exertion, but the fasciae are there to coordinate and dissipate the energy. In addition, they provide a strong point for the muscles and, by virtue of their special viscoelastic properties, absorb and dampen out part of the energy.

Trauma usually occurs in an unexpected way, and the muscular system is thus unprepared to defend against it by absorbing any of the great quantity of energy that is suddenly unleashed on the body. Therefore, it is up to the fasciae to absorb, dampen, and try to channel this energy in different directions in order to attenuate its damaging effects and avoid injury to the organs. When the energy is too great, or concentrated on a very limited area, structures may tear and organs may be damaged.

Studies conducted into the changes in fasciae following injury have shown that their viscoelastic properties can be profoundly changed. Such modifications occur immediately after the critical event, showing that the fasciae have absorbed a significant part of the energy of the accident.

Main Fascial Chains

Given the ubiquity of the fasciae, it could be said that fascial chains are present everywhere in the body. Certainly, if one concentrates on a particular area, it is always possible to identify a fascial chain because it is this unit which acts as the transmission belt for the propagation of force.

However, as we have seen, the major body functions always involve the body acting as a whole. This means that the important chains are far more extensive, linking the entire body from one end to the other. Even at this level, we could describe a large number of different chains. However, anatomical analysis of the fasciae, including the direction and thickness of their fibers, and their collagen content, as well as the more specific function of certain parts of the body compared with others, leads us to believe that certain fascial chains are preferentially brought into play in human mechanics.

We will focus on a few of the most important fascial chains. The transmission of force towards the interior of a fascial chain occurs not only upwards or downwards, but also from the inside towards the outside and vice versa. At crossover points, these chains can even pass from one side of the body to the other. Some of the chains in the trunk mainly function in an oblique direction and therefore also link one side of the body to the other. Obviously, any fascial chain will behave in the same way, whether the energy is ascending or descending.

We will look at a few internal, external, and meningeal chains, although it should always be borne in mind that all such chains are permanently interrelated with one another.

EXTERNAL CHAINS

Starting in the lower limb

Three different fascial chains which start here will be described:

- one lateral
- one anterior
- one posterior

Lateral chain

Starting in the foot, it rises through the following elements (Fig. 6-6):

- the lateral fascia of the leg
- transfer points at the knee and the head of the fibula
- follows the anterolateral surface of the thigh via the iliotibial tract and the fascia lata
- transfer points at the hip and pelvis

Here it meets with a horizontal chain linked to the perineum via the piriformis and internal obturator muscles.

Fig. 6-6   Lateral Chain

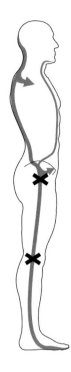

From the pelvis it ascends:

- *either* along an anterior pathway following the rectus abdominis muscle and then the thoracic fasciae
- transfer points at the clavicle
- finally arriving at the lateral cranium via the superficial fascia;
- or along a posterior pathway following the thoracolumbar fascia
- arrives at the posterior part of the scapular girdle, where it forms a transfer point at the scapula
- where it meets with the oblique chain of the scapular girdle through the fasciae of the external rotator muscles of the shoulder
- finally arriving at the posterior part of the base of the skull via the fasciae of the trapezius, splenius, and longissimus capitis muscles

Anterior chain

Starting in the foot, it rises through the following elements (Fig. 6-7):

- the anteromedial fascia of the leg
- forms a transfer point at the medial surface of the knee
- where part of any force can be transmitted to the anterolateral part of the thigh by the oblique fascial fibers
- then follows the fasciae of the adductor muscles
- forms a transfer point at the pubis and the inguinal ligament before rising, like the previous chain, through the rectus abdominis muscle and then possibly passing over to the other side via the fasciae of the oblique muscles

- At the pelvis, it meets with two internal chains:
  — one represented by the fascia iliaca
  — another perineal chain via the superficial perineal fascia

Fig. 6-7 Anterior Chain   **Fig. 6-8** Posterior Chain

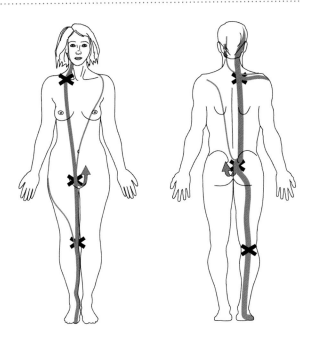

Posterior chain

Starting at the foot (Fig. 6-8):

- follows the posterior fascia of the calf
- forms a transfer point at the knee
- preferentially follows the fascia of the biceps femoris
- forms a transfer point at the buttocks with the ischium, sacrum, coccyx, the sacrotuberous ligament, and then finally at the iliac crest. From there it rises behind in the same way as the external chain, and can also cross over to the other side via the oblique fibers of the thoracolumbar fascia.
- At the buttocks, it meets up with two other chains:
  — one horizontal chain: the perineal chain through the coccyx and the sacrospinous and sacrotuberous ligaments
  — the other, a vertical chain: the dura mater chain through the coccyx and the fibers which are continuous between the dura mater and the sacrotuberous ligament via the sacrum and the coccyx

Starting in the upper limb

We will cover one medial and one lateral chain.

Medial chain

Starting at the hand (*Fig. 6-9*):

- follows the anteromedial edge of the muscles to the medial epichodyle of the humerus
- forms a transfer point at the elbow;
- here, some of the energy can be transmitted into the lateral chain by the oblique fibers of the aponeurosis of the biceps
- follows the medial intermuscular septum
- then extends via the coracobrachial fascia
- forms a transfer point at the acromion and the clavicle
- terminating at the anterolateral cranium via the superficial cervical fascia and the aponeuroses of the scalene muscles

Lateral chain

The lateral chain works most heavily in the upper limb and, as will be discussed later on, it is in this chain that osteopathic help will most often be needed.
    Starting at the wrist (*Fig. 6-9*), the chain follows :

- either the anterolateral edge of the fascia along the radius
- or the posterolateral edge of the same fascia
- forms a transfer point at the lateral surface of the elbow
- follows the lateral intermuscular septum;
- at the deltoid "V," it can continue in two different directions:
  - an anteromedial path via the medial part of the deltoid fascia. Here it transverses along a chain composed of the pectoral fasciae and then follows the same path as the internal chain.
  - or along a posterolateral pathway via the lateral edge of the deltoid fascia, forming a transfer point at the spine of the scapula. Here, it meets up with the posterior oblique chain represented by the fasciae of the latissimus dorsi and the lateral rotator muscles, and finally arrives at the base of the skull by following the same path as the posterior chain.

Internal chains

We will focus on three internal chains:

- one peripheral
- one central
- one mixed

Peripheral chain

We will start with this chain at the perineum, but it should be remembered that it is linked to the external chains through the perineal fascia and those of the piriformis and obturator muscles.
    Starting at the perineum (*Fig. 6-10*):

Fig. 6-9 Medial and Lateral Chains   **Fig. 6-10** Peripheral Chain

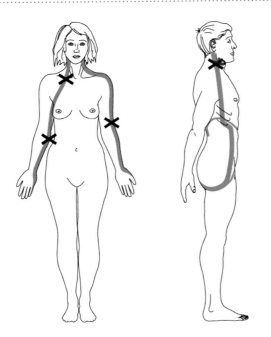

- it continues up through either the transversalis fascia or the peritoneum
- forms a transfer point at the diaphragm
- follows the endothoracic fascia
- arrives at the scapular girdle, where it forms a transfer point
- then follows approximately the same path as the external chains to finish at the base of the skull

It should be noted that the peripheral chains can also pass by the pleurae to arrive at the shoulder at some fasciae above the pleura (sometimes known as the diaphragm of Bourgerey) and from there passes up to the base of the skull like all the other chains.

Central chain

We will start with this chain at the diaphragm, but it should be remembered that below this lies a whole system of supporting fasciae, and that the abdominal fasciae are continuous with the pelvic fasciae.

From the diaphragm, this chain follows:

- the pericardium
- the pharyngobasilar fascia
- at the thoracic outlet, it makes connection with the deep and middle cervical fasciae, and therefore some energy could be redirected towards the supporting bones;
- subsequently, it forms a transfer point at the hyoid bone; here also, the superficial cervical fascia could absorb some energy;

- it then arrives at the base of the skull via the pterygotemporomaxillary and interpterygoid fasciae
- from where it can continue into the dura mater of the brain via nervous extensions which bring it to meet up with the above-mentioned fasciae

Mixed chain

From the perineum, it follows:

- the umbilico-prevesical fascia
- forms a transfer point at the umbilicus
- where it meets the fascia transversalis
- or follows the round ligament of the liver and the falciform ligament
- forms a transfer point at the diaphragm
- from which it follows the same path as either the peripheral or the central chain described above

Meningeal chain

Its lower point of departure is the coccyx, but, as previously noted, it may be influenced by the internal chains, the perineal fasciae, or the external chains which form transfer points at the coccyx, the sacrum, and the pubis (Fig. 6-11).

Fig. 6-11 Meningeal Chain

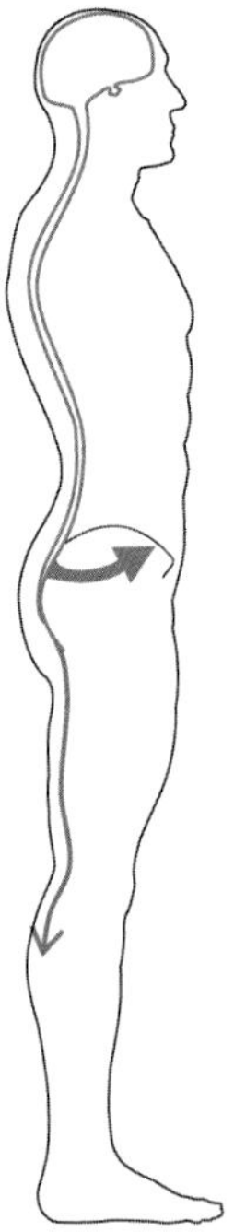

It then rises in the vertebral column where it makes contact with many transfer points with the vertebrae (which serves as a safeguard and back-up system):

- **anterior**: with the common posterior vertebral ligament over the entire length of the column, two transfer points of which are particularly strong:

— the lower part of the coccygeal ligament

— its upper attachment points at C2 and C3;

- **lateral**: the dura mater sends out two lateral meningeal extensions which travel with the nerve as far as the intervertebral foramen. Here, it is strongly attached around the edge of the bone, thereby forming bilateral strong points as well as spinal roots. This prevents over-stretching of the roots and the spinal cord.
- Then it enters the cranial cavity via the foramen magnum, around which it is strongly attached. Inside the cranium, this chain spreads out spherically to attach all over the cranial cavity. The articulations are most pronounced at the base of the skull. In order to guarantee improved mobility and to enhance its protective function, it forms two large septa:

  — the tentorium cerebelli, which provides enhanced horizontal anchoring

  — the falx cerebelli and falx cerebri, which are attached to the crista galli and which provide enhanced sagittal anchoring

It is continuous with the exterior surface of the cranium:

- at its base, through its extensions around the cranial nerves
- over the vault, with the epicranial fasciae via the dural venous sinuses

MAJOR POINTS OF DAMPENING

Fascial chains transmit mobility throughout the body but are also a focus for forces which might disturb their function. So that these forces are not automatically transmitted all along the chain, there are special dampening points distributed throughout each chain. Some of these, located at convergence points, are particularly important (*Fig. 6-12*). We will specifically mention, moving from below upward, the:

- pelvic girdle
- diaphragm
- scapular girdle
- hyoid bone
- occipitocervical junction

Pelvic girdle

Transfer point between the lower limbs and:

- the trunk
- the perineum

This represents a point of convergence for forces, in response to which it is permanently adapting, controlling, and redirecting by virtue of its mobility and architecture. Here, descending, ascending, and transverse (via the internal chain) forces are dampened and dissipated as soon as they reach a critical level.

Fig. 6-12 Points Where Shocks Can Be Absorbed

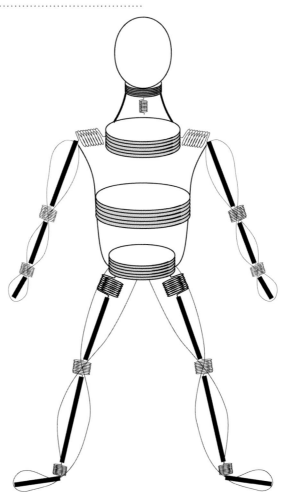

Diaphragm

Apart from its role as the main muscle of respiration, the diaphragm also fulfills other vital functions, mechanical as well as physiological:

- It hermetically separates the thoracic and abdominal cavities, that is, separates a region of negative pressure from one where the pressure steadily rises as one moves in a caudal direction.
- It is subject to pulling forces acting in two different directions:
  - cephalad, because of the thoracic, peripheral, and central fasciae
  - caudal, because of the abdominal fasciae and the weight of the organs it supports.

Despite these opposing forces, to be able to continue to adequately fulfill its functions, it must at all times remain flexible and functional, in which it is aided by the pressure difference. These functions are in:

- respiration
- hemodynamic mobilization
- suspending the abdominal mass
- as a visceral motor which, by virtue of its constant piston motion, keeps the organs moving incessantly, thereby enhancing their capacity to function efficiently

Its anatomical design points to its mechanical function. It is composed of a peripheral muscular portion, which is applied to the internal edge of the thoracic cavity, and which constitutes the diaphragmatic driving force. However, this costal part cannot be attached if the diaphragm is to be perfectly functional in this respect. Therefore, it must be attached elsewhere. It is this function which is looked after by the purely fascial part of the organ, namely, the central tendon.

The central tendon is suspended by a strong fascial sheet, the pericardium, which provides a strong point around which the diaphragm can press in order to open up during inhalation. Its pressure on the abdominal mass is relatively mild in the normal situation, given that the latter is not a strong point and is predisposed to being pushed down and forwards. This is why, as was previously explained, the perineum and the diaphragm work together synergistically and in harmony with one another.

During strenuous exertion, the diaphragm exerts more pressure on the abdominal mass, which is being made rigid by contraction of the abdominal muscles, or contraction of the muscles of both the abdomen and the pelvis at the same time.

Many studies have been conducted to elucidate the mechanics of the diaphragm.

Paiva et al., studying supine patients, showed that the contact between diaphragm and lung is uniform and corresponds to an area which is more or less equal in all subjects, whatever their weight. There is a uniform pressure gradient acting on the diaphragm, and this remains the same whether the subject is at rest or exerting herself, and despite the different organs found on either side. The pressures measured at the diaphragm were 9.7 centimeters of water on the right, and 9.2 on the left.

The radius of curvature of the diaphragm is not even, but instead decreases as the height decreases. When the diaphragm contracts and the volume of the lung increases, the radius decreases with height and it becomes more spherical. It can improve the conversion of tension into pressure when the volume of the lung increases.

Verschakelen et al. measured the displacement of the diaphragm during exhalation and found that the readings increased from front to back with 100% behind, 90% in the middle, and 60% in front.

Movement of the diaphragm is coupled with that of the ribs and the abdominal musculature. The correlation is closer with its median and posterior parts. The posterior part is especially closely coupled with displacement of the abdominals.

During normal inhalation, the diaphragm shortens, with the shortening of the posterior part usually being more marked than that of the anterior part. After phrenicotomy, Decramer et al. showed that the posterior part elongates during inhalation, while the anterior part elongates in some animals and shortens in others.

On the subject of the diaphragm, let us pause one moment to consider its innervation because this can certainly explain certain lesional patterns seen in the cervicoscapular region (Figs. 6-13 & 6-14).

Fig. 6-13   Embryonic Diaphragm (after Langman/Sadler)

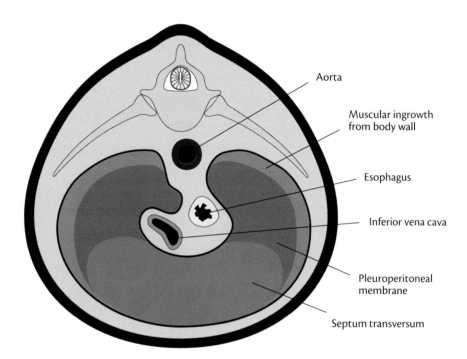

Initially located in the cervical myotome, the transverse septum which will develop into the diaphragm steadily migrates downward during embryogenesis to eventually assume its definitive position. Supplied from the beginning by the phrenic nerve, it travels downward together with it. During its migration, the phrenic nerve does not simply follow the diaphragm, but also sends out numerous collateral fibers all the way. These collateral nerves will go on to innervate other structures, including the:

- thymus
- pericardium
- parietal pleura
- superior and inferior vena cava
- perivascular fibrous capsules (Glisson's capsules)
- trigeminal ganglia

Fig. 6-14   Development of the Embryonic Diaphragm at Week 5 (after Langman/Sadler)

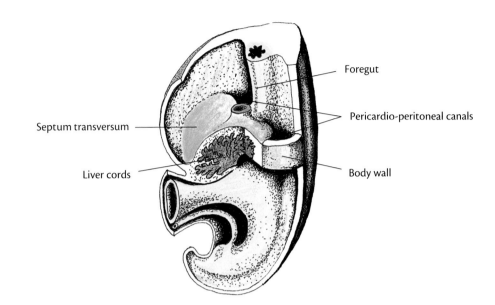

Foregut

Pericardio-peritoneal canals

Septum transversum

Body wall

Liver cords

It also anastomoses with cranial nerves X and XII, the subclavian nerve, and the cervical sympathetics. Therefore, it is easy to understand its importance and why the scapular girdle is often the focus for incomprehensible problems. The neuronal channel constituted by the phrenic nerve often explains such problems.

To finish, it should be noted that the diaphragm represents an important point inside the thorax for the dampening of mechanical forces transmitted by the fasciae, and also for attenuating pressure variations.

Scapular girdle

All the fasciae—both internal and external—converge and form a transfer point at the scapular girdle. This is a very hard-working area and is very likely to suffer in the event of any kind of fascial dysfunction. This region must be constantly controlling and adjusting to compensate for work being done lower down in regions which are relatively rigid, and higher up in regions which are hypermobile.

The scapular girdle must permanently perform a balancing act to harmonize all the forces which converge there, and thereby protect the vital areas which are located both above and below it. Moreover, attached to it is another hypermobile segment, namely, the upper limb, which represents the most hard-working area of the body, in mechanical terms. It is also a focus for vertical, oblique, and transverse forces.

For all of these reasons, the architecture of this region is very specialized, oriented towards hypermobility. It is the only region, apart from the sternoclavicular junction, where the anchor points are exclusively created by soft tissues.

The convergence of internal, external, ascending, and descending forces provides an explanation for why the cervicoscapular junction is so often the site of restrictions.

Hyoid bone

The central pericardium-pharyngobasilar fascial chain has points of peripheral transfer, the pericardial ligaments, and connections with the middle and deep cervical fasciae, but they are not as important as those of the scapular girdle. Still, serious tension due to major forces could be transmitted suddenly into the base of the skull, with potential danger to intracranial structures.

To avoid this situation, a special structure is interposed at the top of this fascial chain, namely, the hyoid bone. Completely suspended by bands of muscular, fascial tissue, the hyoid bone floats in all spatial planes, held in place by its attachments to the mandible, mastoid bone, styloid process, scapula, and thyroid cartilage.

The central fascial chain forms a transfer point at the end of the pharyngobasilar fascia at the hyoid bone, after which it continues up via the interptyeryoid et pterygotemporomaxillary fasciae.

The hyoid bone, apart from its role in fixing the thyroid cartilage for vocalization, is also present in order to dampen and distribute force traveling in the central chain, either in an anterolateral direction via the superficial cervical fascia, or in a posterior direction towards the temporal bone via the digastric muscle and Riolan's bouquet.

Occipitocervical junction

The cranial 'sphere' posed on its occipital support constitutes a point of convergence between all the descending cervicocranial chains and the underlying chains. This point of convergence is also relevant to forces traveling in the intracranial chains and the vertebral dura mater chain, which form a transfer point here.

Therefore, it represents a particularly hard-working region, which explains the numerous muscles which control it, long or short, in order to adapt it constantly to all the possible variations in tension, with the aim of protecting, as effectively as possible, the central 'computer' and its information-conducting extensions.

All the fasciae are inserted around its edge. It represents the first descending and the last ascending shock absorber. Thus, the transmission of forces into the cranial cavity is inhibited. In addition, inside the cranial cavity, there is a whole system of buffering membranes to mitigate any excess energy which passes this barrier. It should be remembered that, in the cranium and in the spinal cord, a hydraulic system is in place there as a back-up for the membrane protection. The frequent demands made of the occipitocervical junction explain why this region is so often a site of restricted mobility.

LESIONAL CHAINS

These represent the path which membranous tensions can follow to propagate over a long distance. There is, in practice, an infinite number of different potential pathways along which damaging chain reactions could propagate, but experience has taught us that such sequences tend to follow certain patterns which, in general, correspond to the fascial chains discussed in the previous section. These lesional chains are therefore distortions – fascial chains which have been perturbed so that they have become dysfunctional. Instead of harmoniously distributing movements and excess energy, these chains have been converted into areas of restriction that are a source of irritation and inhibited mobility.

Many different factors can trigger a damaging chain reaction, including trauma (e.g., a sprain, a fall directly onto the coccyx, or a direct blow on an area of soft tissue), scars, infection, inflammation, and emotional stress. Such factors can induce a point of fascial dysfunction which, if uncorrected, can compromise the quality of the tissue and may, with time, propagate all along the fascial chain to give rise to dysfunction in the future. The secondary problem may actually manifest far from the site of the primary point of dysfunction. A lesional chain can start anywhere and can travel either a very short distance or very far, for example, a primary problem in the foot can eventually manifest at the occipitocervical junction or even in the cranium.

All injuries do not necessarily induce a damaging chain reaction. Sometimes a reaction will appear soon after the original trauma, whereas other times, it can take weeks or even months to manifest. This will depend on a number of factors:

- the seriousness of the original injury
- the age of the patient
- the capacity of the patient to adapt and compensate

Obviously, the younger the patient, the better the body will be able to defend itself.

A healthy, physiologically functional body will do all in its power to attenuate the effects of a lesion or localized restriction, and will attempt to dissipate any excess energy by distributing it across as wide an area as possible.

With advancing age (and the necessary concomitant accumulation of a history of insults), the body will become less and less competent at defending itself against the effects of such lesions, its capacities for compensation and adaptation will diminish, and, if the force is too great, the system will be overwhelmed and a damaging chain reaction may become established. This may have extremely serious consequences.

It should be remembered that the tissues retain a record of all the injuries they have suffered and that, whatever their nature, these accumulate and, at some time, will inevitably be recalled by the body.

Temporal traumatic summation is far from being an absolute rule. Certain people develop dysfunction rapidly, while others continue for years—even forever in some cases—with no problems whatsoever. This depends on the individual's inherent 'vitality' and capacity to deal with the constraints of life.

An important factor when it comes to limiting the spread of a lesion is the dampening areas, which are many in number and distributed throughout the body. Dampening structures include adipose tissue, hydraulic systems (e.g., the cerebrospinal fluid), special architectural configurations, and joints.

Gradually over time, as one dampening system is worn out, the force is transferred onto the next one. It will be inhibited at the major points of dampening, identified in a previous section, but, once these in turn have been overwhelmed, it will finally reach its target and there mediate its deleterious effects. It is obvious that, when a propagating chain reaction encounters an existing weak point (an articular, tissular, or visceral weak point), it will accelerate the rate of degeneration there.

A lesional chain can start in any part of the body and, from there, spread either upwards or downwards. The direction depends on exactly where it started, factors related to the forces involved, and the person's capacity to compensate and adapt. Therefore, we must consider ascending and descending chain reactions.

Descending chain reactions

Most of these occur, in order of importance, in the cranium, the cervical vertebrae, the scapular girdle, the pelvis, the lower limbs, the thorax, the diaphragm, and the abdomen. We will describe some of the more frequently encountered examples, bearing in mind that their pathways are usually determined by the pattern of the relevant fascial chain.

- Starting from a restriction in the epicranial fascia, a descending chain reaction can become established through the superficial cervical fascia down to the scapular girdle or, beyond that, down through the upper thorax or the upper limb.
- If the point of departure is at the base of the skull (in the broad sense) or intracranial, it could be conducted by the deep cervical fascia and the aponeuroses of the scalene muscles to rejoin the path of the previously mentioned reaction.
- If the restriction is located in the mediastinum or the thorax, the perturbation may eventually reach the abdominal fasciae or as far as the true pelvis.
- Finally, if the perturbation is at the level of the psoas muscle, the perineum, or the short muscles of the hip, the chain reaction may propagate downwards, eventually causing a problem in the knee or even the ankle.

It will be noticed that descending chain reactions travel less far than the fascial chains described above—it is rare to encounter a primary problem in the head giving rise to a secondary problem in the foot, although this can occur.

Ascending chain reactions

Ascending chain reactions are more common than descending ones, no doubt due to the fact that the constant pressure on the ground which is necessary for our stability, together with our constant battle against gravity and the fact that our organs are in a state of suspension, all mean that most of the mechanical work we are obliged to do involves traction in a downward direction.

In contrast to descending chain reactions, ascending ones often propagate over long distances. We will cover a few common examples here.

The most common chain reaction which starts at the foot transmits along the lateral chain. Following a sprained ankle, traction on the external fascia can have effects at the head of the fibula or at the external part of the knee and generate functional pain at those foci.

If the lesional chain continues to ascend, it can cause disturbance in the hip (and then in the true pelvis via the fasciae of the piriformis and internal obturator muscles) and then in the sacroiliac joint. From there, it can spread via the thoracolumbar fascia or the latissimus dorsi muscle to the shoulder. Finally, if its spread is not curtailed, it may finish in the cervical vertebrae or the cranium. Of course, as noted, its point of departure can be located anywhere from the knee upwards.

A direct fall onto the coccyx can trigger a damaging chain reaction in the dura mater which can spread, from element to element, as far as the intracranial membranes.

A problem in the perineum can be transmitted by either the abdominal viscera or by the transversalis fascia. Transferring at the diaphragm, it can continue on up via the pleural system or the endothoracic fascia to reach the scapular girdle and, ultimately, the cervical vertebrae or the cranium.

Next we will consider the example of a damaging chain reaction that we have encountered several times and which, at first impression, would seem to be more theoretical than real. It can start in either the bladder or the umbilico-prevesical fascia and continue successively via the round ligament, the falciform ligament, the diaphragm, and the pericardium to reach the pharyngobasilar fascia, where it manifests as a throat problem.

A patient consulted recently for a sore throat and painful swallowing. This woman had recently undergone an endoscopic procedure and had a scar near her median umbilical ligament. Pressure on this scar was found to exacerbate her throat symptoms. The scar was the point of departure for an ascending chain reaction which resulted in pain in the throat. The patient's throat problem was resolved by correcting a restriction that was located affecting the median umbilical ligament.

This is far from an isolated example, and it underlines the reality of fascial chains and the fact that they can propagate lesions. It is often vital to extend the field of investigation to remote parts of the body in order to gain a full understanding of a particular problem.

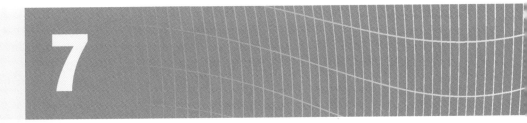

Fascial Tests

The Purpose of the Tests

The fasciae represent a sensitive receptor system which is prone to different forms of perturbation in everyday life. Such disturbances can be due to:

- trauma
- obstetrical problems
- poor posture
- surgery (scarring, adhesions)
- inflammation
- accidents
- tension, bad postural habits (usually occupation-related)
- false movements
- stress

These insults will induce biochemical changes in the connective tissue which will, in turn, have effects on its viscoelastic properties and thereby its very structure. Its density will increase, the collagen fibers will tend to align along the axis of the lines of force, and the tissue will lose elasticity. All such changes in the fasciae can be detected and assessed by palpation, and can sometimes even be seen directly with the eye.

The purpose of a fascial test is to use the exquisite sensitivity of our hands to detect a variety of problems which might be affecting the underlying tissues, in order to obtain information to orient and guide the choice of therapeutic modalities.

Test Methods

Fascial restrictions are detected using the hands. It could be said that testing is based on applying one fascial system to another: one with problems being listened to by another in order to sense and understand those problems.

We have already discussed the idea of 'fascial memory,' which represents the recording of an impression of the various traumas (in the broadest sense) experienced by an individual. Our purpose is to detect these impressions and, if possible, to resolve or at least attenuate them.

As we have seen, the fasciae are endowed with a contractile mechanism by virtue of their innervation, which is derived during development. This mechanism induces minute but constant movement with a periodicity of between eight and fourteen cycles per minute. In addition, the fasciae act as ropes and pulleys in the transmission of forces. These observations have led us to develop two distinct types of tests:

- listening tests
- mobility tests

These two types of tests are not mutually exclusive. In fact, a listening test is just a special type of mobility test in which the actual movement is simply an extremely small one—not induced or even visible, but rather sensed. Those tests referred to as mobility tests involve, as the name indicates, a much larger movement, one which is visible and which generates tension at some point.

Listening Tests

A listening test involves placing a hand on some part of the body in order to detect any underlying changes. The hand must be kept perfectly passive in a receptive mode so that it can detect extremely small movements. Investigations into the sensitivity of the hand have shown that it can detect movements as small as ten microns in amplitude. A difference of only five per cent was found between measurements made by the hands and those recorded using a sophisticated apparatus.

TEST PROTOCOL

A listening test requires certain elementary precautions, without which its results are worthless. Obviously, a listening test cannot be undertaken by anyone at any time—efficacy requires an enormous amount of practice as well as the confidence on the part of the practitioner that a hand can indeed detect such tiny movements. The validity of the results of the test depend on:

- the manual contact
- the practitioner being in harmony with the patient
- the neutrality of the practitioner

Manual contact

Given that the amplitude of the movements to be detected is of the order of a few microns, it is obvious that even the tiniest grain of sand could invalidate the results of the test.

The first precaution is to ensure that your hands are not too cold, for this would provoke a guarding reaction. The hand should be placed flat on the area to be investigated, with as great an area of contact with the patient's tissues as possible. This is done for two reasons:

- The greater the area of contact, the greater the number of receptors stimulated, and therefore the greater the amount of information collected.
- The flatter the hand, the easier it will be to obtain accurate information about the underlying fasciae.

Above all, contact with the finger tips is to be avoided. The tissues are exquisitely sensitive and if palpation is too aggressive, nothing will be heard, just silence. This is because it often does not take much to induce a reflex spasm.

The pressure applied should be very moderate. If the pressure is too great, the level of listening that is desired will be exceeded and you will no longer be able to perceive movement. Remember that the most important receptors in this context are the pressure receptors in your hand.

The hand must rest gently on the surface of the skin, exerting only its natural weight. At the same time, the two skin surfaces should be in firm contact, as if you were trying to create a sucker effect. The hand is 'stuck' to the tissues to make it easier to feel their motility.

Harmony with the patient

A listening test represents the most fine type of palpation. The tissues have a memory of what happened to them in the past, and the purpose of the listening test is to access this information and understand the patient's history. The dialog is a passive one: the patient is unaware of the information being transmitted to the osteopath from their fasciae; it is at the same level as their unconscious. If the practitioner fails to establish a good 'rapport' with the patient, there will be no exchange of information in the other direction.

The patient and their tissues must be treated with respect, and we should act as if we were asking permission to establish a dialog with the tissues.

Neutrality of the practitioner

All tests should be conducted in a spirit of complete neutrality in order to guarantee efficacy. The practitioner should not have any preconceived ideas and should remain perfectly passive, just tuned in and listening.

It is the patient's rhythm which is important. If the practitioner's rhythm is imposed on the patient in any way, there will be no response, or the response detected will be misleading. This aspect is not so easy for those untrained in this type of palpation. If the motility takes some time to manifest, an inexperienced practitioner will tend to project their own rhythm into the patient's tissues, with the result that the practitioner is simply detecting their own motion.

All of the practitioner's attention should be focused exclusively on the contact zone and he or she should be guided only by the underlying tissues. This will require complete awareness and full concentration because the response, when it comes, will be rapid.

It is only when all these requirements have been met that the test proper can begin. Only in this way will the tissues be in a position to communicate with the practitioner and reveal their perturbations, problems, and history.

Once you have learned how to properly listen to the patient, it is surprising how quickly the tissues begin to 'talk.' The sooner that mutual confidence is established, the sooner there will be a response. At this point, you will have the impression of movements with a much greater amplitude, as if the fact of being in harmony with the patient amplifies the tiny movements being assessed.

However, a short lapse of concentration or some sudden movement by the practitioner can bring the dialog to an abrupt end. It does not take very long to test the motility of a tissue, although if the basic rules are not adhered to, it is quite possible to spend hours in contact with a tissue without deriving any information whatsoever.

LISTENING TESTS

The purpose of a listening test is to detect abnormalities in soft tissues. Since abnormality can only be defined in terms of normality, we will now try to define what constitutes the normal, insofar as there is such a thing.

Norm

The norm encompasses a number of different factors which can be immediately assessed with the hand:

- The *temperature* of the tissue. Although different parts of the skin can have a different temperature, only a certain range is normal. In assessing temperature, the practitioner must sometimes compare the temperature of the patient's skin with their own, or with some other part of the patient's body.

It is common to detect a higher temperature than the normal threshold as a result of a reaction in the underlying tissue. Sometimes, especially in the feet and hands, temperatures which are below the lower threshold of normalcy are also encountered.

- The *texture* of the tissue. The tissue should be yielding—neither too tight nor too loose—and should be pleasant to the touch. It should give easily and be elastic, that is, regain its original shape after it is depressed. The tissue's normal elasticity will depend on the specific fascia under consideration.

- The mobility of the tissue. Although certain tissues tend to have a preferred direction of movement (discussed more later), in general, the mobility of a tissue may be considered normal when it is mobile in all spatial planes. When the hand is placed on the tissue, you should get an impression of floating in all the spatial planes, as if your hand were resting on a soft surface which is floating on a basin filled with water. No one direction should be preferred to another, and, if the surface is actively displaced, the underlying tissue should follow without resistance.
- The rhythm of the tissues. It has already been pointed out that the tissues pulse rhythmically, with a frequency of between eight and fourteen cycles per minute. In the vast majority of cases, a rhythm that is faster or slower than this can be considered abnormal. However, it should be borne in mind that some people might have a faster or slower rhythm without there being an abnormality.

It is also important to know that this rhythm can change depending on the patient's condition at a certain time. Rhythm is especially easy to detect in certain parts of the body, notably, the anterior part of the lower limbs, the thorax, and the skull. On the other hand, there are parts of the body where it is very difficult or even impossible to detect, including the posterior side of the thigh, the buttocks, on the back, and over the abdomen. (A small digression about the abdomen: Although it is difficult to feel the rhythm of the superficial fascia, it is relatively easy to bypass this layer and assess the rhythm of the various underlying fascial elements deeper down.)

The human body sometimes presents us with contradictions which are real, even if they are completely incomprehensible.

Standing listening tests

Initially, it is common to perform a test with:

- the patient in an erect, standing position, with their legs slightly apart, head pointed forwards, and eyes closed
- the practitioner behind the patient with their hand gently on the patient's head, but exerting no pressure

In this position, a particular type of movement of the body is often detected in the form of forward bending, sidebending, or backward bending. The fact of having established a stationary point on the skull creates a connection between the floor and the head, and all the fasciae between these two points are going to be able to move as long as they have such a fixed point. For this reason, the body may incline in an entirely involuntary fashion, with the fixed point acting as a focal point for the tensions which induce flexion of the body towards it.

This can reveal both that there is an underlying problem, as well as something about the context of the problem, although no formal diagnosis can be made on the basis of this test alone, as it is a screen.

This is a perfect example of how fascial dynamics affect the overall mechanics of the body. When performing this type of test in patients who are depressed (in whom the fasciae are usually affected), one must be especially attentive because these patients have a tendency to fall backwards—be ready to support them.

Listening tests for the lower limbs

The general method for all listening tests involves placing the hand on a certain region of the body with a view to detecting underlying abnormality. It is also possible to place the two hands at some distance apart and feel if the motility which establishes itself between the two points is normal or not.

After years of experience, and with particularly exquisite sensitivity, the ultimate goal is to be able to place one or both hands on any part of the body and detect a center of tension anywhere else in the body. This is not a minor ambition—some achieve it, but it must be admitted that they are rare.

To come back to the lower limbs, we are now going to cover the protocol for the various tests with its variations: the patient, of course, is supine and completely relaxed.

Place the hands flat on the dorsal side of the feet: feel whether movement is harmonious or whether there seems to be any tendency to pull in a specific direction. Such pulling would indicate a pathological axis: a change in organization in connective tissue due to some trauma (of any kind) has created a preferred vector of nonphysiological movement. Subsequently, the tension should be followed back, step by step, until the precise starting point is identified.

In order to confirm what you feel passively, shift the hand ever so slightly—more as if you were about to shift it, or thinking of shifting it, rather than actually shifting it. If the shift is in the direction of the center of tension, no resistance will be offered. On the other hand, if the movement is in the wrong direction, straight away you will feel tension opposing the movement.

The modalities and principles underlying motility tests are the same for all parts of the body and therefore do not require further description. All listening tests are performed with the patient in a supine position. We prefer to start at the foot and move upward towards the pelvis in a step-by-step manner.

Listening to the ankle

Place one hand on the dorsal side of the foot, and the other on the lower edge of the tibia. In a normal situation, you should feel movement between the two hands which harmonizes in all spatial planes, as if you were manipulating a sphere.

Listening to the knee

Place one hand over the tibial condyles, and the other on the lower part of the femur, excluding the patella. In a normal situation, lateral, superior, and inferior translation should be free, as should rotations, with the latter often dominant (Fig. 7-1).

Fig. 7-1   Listening to the Knee

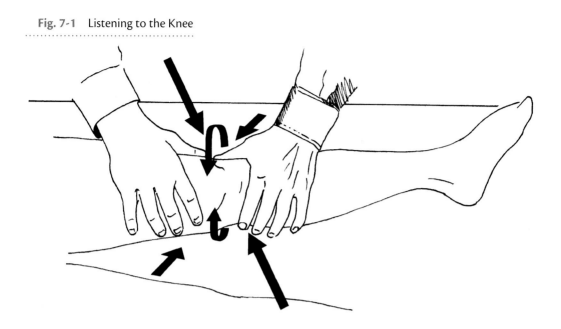

Listening to the thigh and lower leg

Place one hand flat in the middle of the thigh, and the other on the anterior, lateral side of the tibia. The cephalad hand should feel internal and external rotation, with the former being dominant. External rotation should dominate in the caudal hand (Fig. 7-2).

Fig. 7-2   Listening to the Thigh and Leg

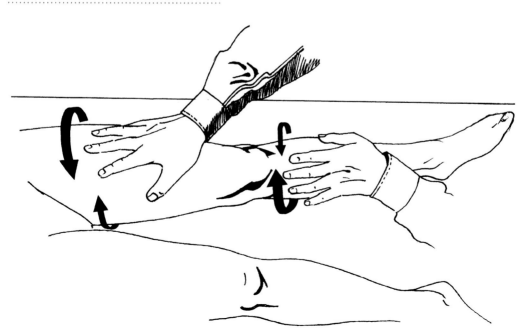

We have seen that the fasciae of the lower limb are composed of fibers running in different directionsin the linked thigh-leg mechanism, it is the medially oblique fibers which predominate in the thigh, and laterally oblique fibers in the lower leg.

Listening to the entire lower limb

The practitioner takes up a position to the side of the patient, facing cephalad. Place one hand flat on the anterolateral side of the lower part of the thigh. Feel movement of the whole lower limb, with external rotation predominant. In fact, the anterior external parts of all the fasciae are thicker and stronger. This listening test can be performed on both sides (Fig. 7-3).

Fig. 7-3   Listening to the Entire Lower Limb

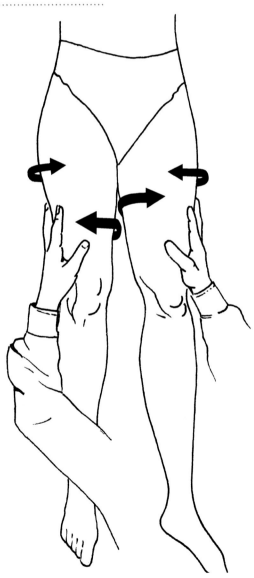

Listening tests for the upper limbs

As previously mentioned, listening tests for the upper limbs are more tricky than those for the lower limbs. In some cases, a listening test cannot even be successfully performed in this region. The difficulty is due to the special features of the upper limbs, which would seem to be connected in parallel, rather than in series, to the rest of the body. If your hand is placed on the dorsal surface of the patient's hand in the normal manner, the sensation of motility is significantly less than in the lower limb—and the situation is the same with local listening tests.

Listening to the arm and forearm

Place one hand on the external anterior surface of the arm below the deltoid 'V,' and the other below the elbow fold over the epicondyle muscles. Use the cephalad hand to feel a movement with external rotation predominant; the caudal hand will feel a movement with internal rotation predominant (Fig. 7-4).

Fig. 7-4   Listening to the Arm and Forearm

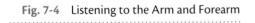

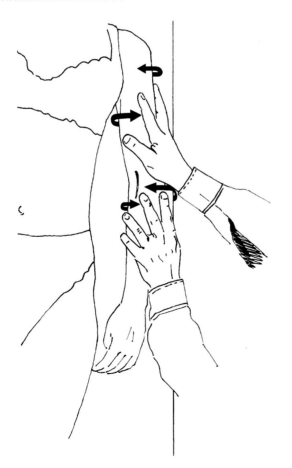

Listening to the entire upper limb

The practitioner takes up a position at the side of the patient, facing cephalad. One hand is placed over the elbow joint at the inferior part of the humerus, where the predominant movement will be internal rotation. This listening test can be performed on both sides simultaneously (Fig. 7-5).

Fig. 7-5   Listening to the Entire Upper Limb Bilaterally

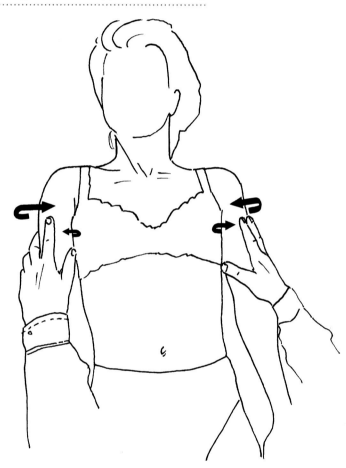

Is this due to the powerful chest muscles and their associated fasciae pulling the upper limb into internal rotation? We have already mentioned the natural tendency of the upper part of the body towards internal rotation. Therefore, it would appear that, in terms of the direction of its motility, the behavior of the upper limb is exactly opposite that of the lower limb. Could this be to establish a general equilibrium and thereby to create functional balance?

Listening tests for the abdomen

Here, we are not going to consider in detail all the possible listening tests for the abdomen—this has been covered already in many other texts, including *Visceral*

Manipulation II by Jean-Pierre Barral. Rather, we will simply point out the difficulties encountered in this region.

The main difficulty is related to the large number of structures which are encountered under the hand, including the peritoneum, the fasciae, the ligaments, the mesenteries, and the organs themselves. Another difficulty is the depth of palpation—how many layers there are between the superficial fascia and the renal fascia!

The general principle with respect to the abdomen is to place the hand flat around the umbilicus and feel for any tension. In order to narrow down the diagnosis, it may be necessary to move the hand in the direction of any perceived tension to pin down its origin as closely as possible.

In the normal situation, the motility of the abdomen is similar to that of all the other tissues, that is, the hand should float over the abdominal cavity with freedom in all spatial planes.

Listening tests for the thorax

The thorax is a region in which the tissue is particularly motile. The difficulty is in distinguishing between the superficial and the deeper tissues, where there are two major fascial systems, namely, the pericardium and the pleurae. In addition, in the lower thorax, there is the diaphragm.

The patient should be in a supine position, with the practitioner positioned at the head.

Lower part of the thorax

Spread the hands wide open on the sides of the thorax, with the fingers following the ribs posteriorly, and the thumbs pointed medially. Test the thorax as a whole, and then make a side-to-side comparison. In a normal person, this elastic cylinder should seem to be able to move around in all planes without any blockage.

An alternative method has the practitioner by the side of the patient and facing cephalad (Fig. 7-6).

Upper part of the thorax

This region is especially difficult because of the presence, in addition to the superficial fasciae, of the pericardium, the dome of the pleura, and the fasciae which are continuous with the scapular girdle.

▶ TWO-HAND TEST (FIG. 7-7)

With both hands wide open on the sides of the thorax, and the base of the hands placed just below the clavicle, spread the fingers to cover the pectoral muscles and point the thumbs in a medial direction. In the normal situation, the movement felt under the hands should be harmonious. If there are tensions present, these may be:

• in the medial direction, if the problem is in the superficial fascia directly over the sternum

- in the medial direction, but with the hand feeling as if it is sinking, if the problem is in or around the pericardium
- in the vertical direction, if the problem is located in the pleural dome
- in the superolateral direction, if the problem involves the periscapular region

Fig. 7-6   Listening to the Lower Thorax

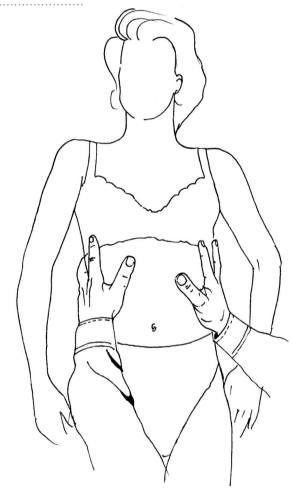

▶ STERNAL TEST

Experience has shown that problems of the upper thorax tend to be focused in the sternum or nearby. This test is done by placing one hand covering the entire sternum, with the base of the hand at the sternal notch. If the hand is in close enough contact with the skin (as if it were a sucker), the motility of the sternal fasciae and those below can be sensed.

The sternum can be conceived as an inverted sacrum being held in the hand. Tiny displacements of the hand can be made to induce the sternum to 'travel' through all the spatial planes, helping us to identify any point of resistance.

Fig. 7-7 Listening to the Upper Thorax

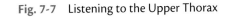

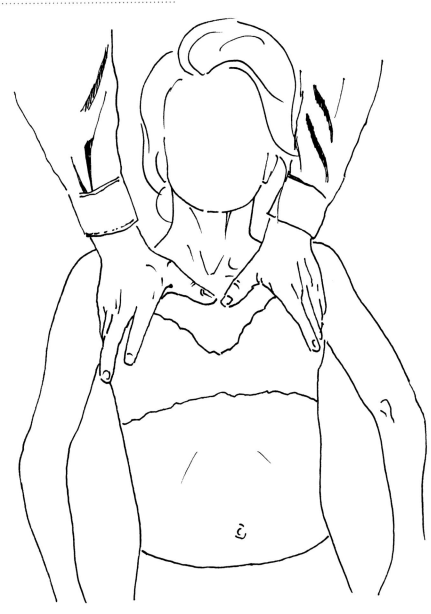

Listening tests for the scapular girdle

For these tests the patient is always supine. The practitioner should be seated behind the patient's head, with the thumbs on the anterior edge of the trapezius muscles near the transverse process of C7. This allows the open hands to rest on the pleural dome, the clavicles, and the root of the shoulder (Fig. 7-8). The thumbs will register any resistance around the first rib, while the hands will register resistance affecting the fascial insertions around the clavicle or tension around the joints.

Some left-right imbalance is common. In right-handed people, the right clavicle shoulder complex can have a slight tendency to point forwards and inside. Of course, a similar phenomenon is seen on the left-hand side of those who are left-handed. If this tendency is too pronounced, impairment of function can result.

Fig. 7-8   Listening to the Entire Shoulder Girdle

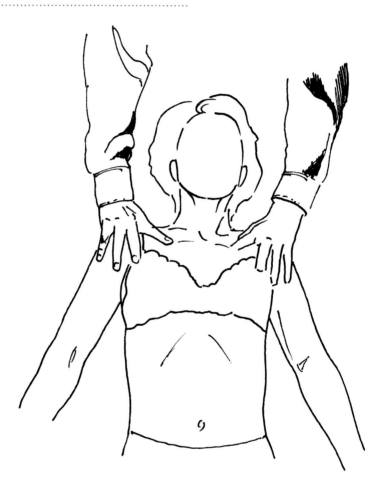

Listening tests for the pelvis

This region contains the articulation point between the powerful lumbosacral fasciae and those of the lower limb, including various strong ligaments, notably the sacrotuberous. Moreover, it contains all the structures in the various cavities of the true pelvis.

Finally, there is the terminal insertion of the dura mater into the sacrum. This gives an idea of the diversity of information available in this region—although its sheer volume can sometimes make the results of a listening test difficult to interpret.

For these tests the patient should be prone. The practitioner should take up a position by the side of the patient, facing cephalad. One hand covers the sacrum like a 'sucker,' with its base covering the inferior lateral angles of the bone (Fig. 7-8).

Fig. 7-8   Listening to the Pelvis

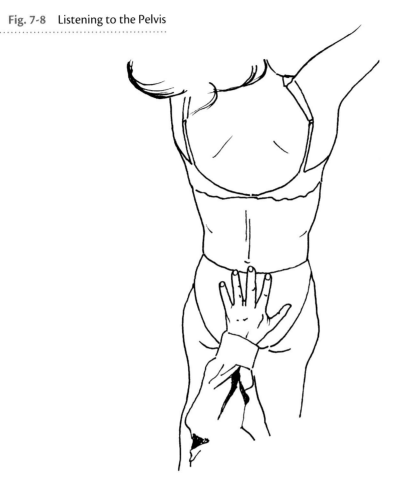

If all is well, the sacrum should be floating harmoniously between the hips. There are a number of common positive findings:

- If the fingers are pulled cephalad, the problem probably resides in the lumbosacral junction or the lumbar fasciae.
- I the base of the hand is pulled towards the feet, the problem may be affecting the coccyx or the sacrotuberous ligament.
- If the hand tends to sink down between the hip bones, the possibility of restrictions in the true pelvis should be considered.
- If the hand is pulled to one side, the problem could be located at the sacroiliac joint, the sacrospinous ligament, or even the ligaments of the hip, pelvis, or trochanter.
- Finally, if the base of the hand is pulled towards the table and cephalad, the possibility of abnormal tension in the dura mater should be considered.

Listening tests for the thoracic fasciae

With the patient prone and the practitioner at their side facing cephalad, either place both hands on either side of the vertebral axis, or just one hand covering the spine and the surrounding area (Fig. 7-9).

Motility is difficult to sense in the lower thoracic region—positive responses are usually indicative of distortion. It is much easier to sense higher up on the back. To feel here, place both hands on the scapulas. Very soon, their movement becomes evident, as if they were floating over the thoracic cavity. The position of the scapulas with respect to the thorax seems to result in amplification of the movement. In the event of distortion, the scapula will tend to be pulled towards the location of the problem.

Fig. 7-9 Listening to the Thoracic Fasciae

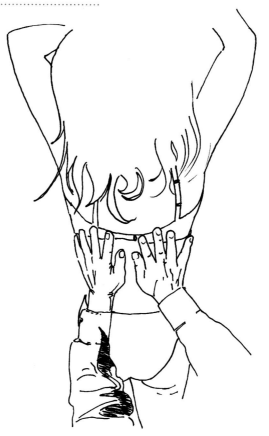

Listening tests for the cranium

In this region, there are several different parameters that can be tested. This complicates the diagnostic process. The following must all be taken into account:

- the intracranial membranes
- the exocranial membranes and the cervical fasciae which are continuous with them

- the spinal meninges
- elements of the central fascial axis

The patient should be supine, regardless of which fascia is being evaluated.

Intracranial membranes

We do not intend to go into detail concerning cranial techniques. We find the standard five-finger hold perfectly suited for a general cranial listening test. If distortion is detected, this can be a followed up with a falx cerebelli technique.

- Support the posterior part of the head with the palm of the left hand, and with the thumb and ring finger pointing out to cover the tentorium cerebelli.
- Place the other hand over the vault, with the middle finger pointing in a sagittal direction along the falx cerebelli.

One of the problems associated with accessing the intracranial membranes is the presence of the exocranial fasciae and the bony structures between them and the hand. As previously discussed, the interior and exterior of the cranium are in communication and therefore can influence one another. For effective intracranial listening, one must 'project' oneself inside the skull.

Exocranial membranes and their extensions

The position is the same as above. Obviously, as the external fasciae of the skull are subject to problems, they should not be ignored. If any superficial tension is detected, the point of resistance should be identified because such a point is extremely disruptive with respect to cranial and cervicoscapular mechanics, as will be discussed later.

We have already mentioned how fascial tension can begin at the base of the skull, especially involving the cervical fasciae. If the lesion is ascending, it will cause a restriction in cranial motility. This is particularly true for the aponeuroses of the sternocleidomastoid muscles and, to an even greater extent, for those of the posterior superficial cervical fascia, which tend to involve the temporal bone in the pathological process.

When the skull is taken into the hand, the hand will be pulled in a caudal direction along the axis of the problematic fibers.

Spinal meninges

Place your hands over the posterior base of the skull, with the fingers crossed over one another in the form of a very shallow 'V.' Then induce a very mild traction following the longitudinal axis of the spine. One you have engaged the tissues, slightly increase the degree of traction to steadily descend as far as the sacrum (Figs. 7-10 & 7-11).

The dura mater is firmly attached at C2 and C3 and also, via radicular extensions, around both sides of the intervertebral foramina. These attachments are not purely theoretical—the dura mater is solidly anchored to the vertebral periosteum to enhance protection of the spinal cord and the nerve roots. We did anatomical investigations into these anchors using pigs and found that tremendous force was necessary to pull them out.

In the normal situation, light traction on the dura mater elicits no response. Since the dura mater is not extensible, any focus of restriction will be easy to feel because it will no longer float free in its bony channel. With a little practice, it is easy to diagnose resistance in any direction along the dura mater.

Fig. 7-10   Position of Hands for Testing the Meninges   **Fig. 7-11**   Spinal Meninges Test

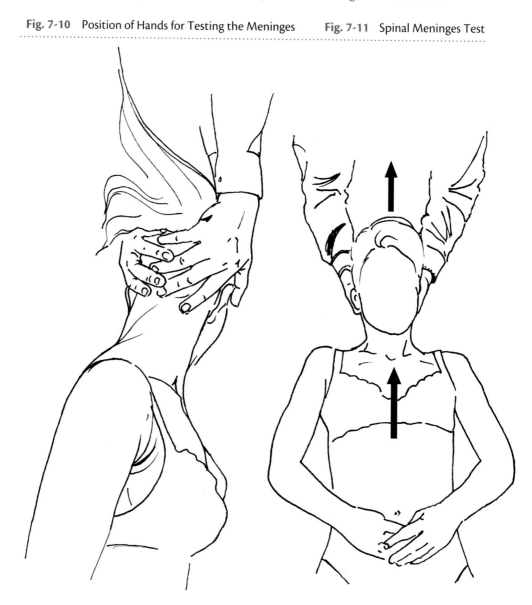

Central fascial axis

The central fascial axis begins around the edges of the foramen magnum. When there is a restriction along the length of the axis, any problem anywhere which involves it will transmit an effect to the base of the cranium.

The hand position for listening to this axis is the same as that for the spinal meninges, described above. The thumbs are directed towards the angle of the mandible (Fig. 7-12).

In the normal situation, this axis is completely free. If there is a problem, two phenomena will be observed:

- Palpatory: The hands will be pulled in a caudal direction, with the skull moving according to the rhythm of the patient's breathing.
- Visual: Looking along the central axis, you should see a rhythmic movement that goes up and down the longitudinal axis of the body. If there is severe restriction that involves the pericardium and diaphragm, the visceral part of the neck, made up of the various cartilages, will sink down into the thorax by a matter of centimeters.

Fig. 7-12   Central Fascial Axis Test

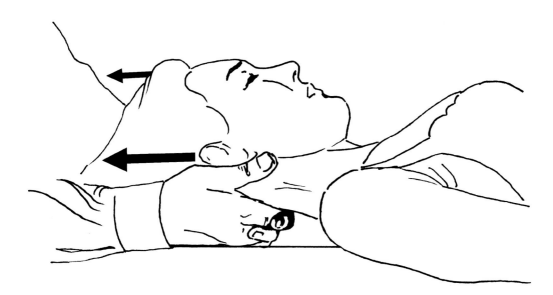

Anteroposterior listening tests

The patient should be supine. The practitioner is positioned at the patient's head, cradling the base of the skull with one hand, and eliciting light traction. The other hand is placed flat over the sternum (Fig. 7-13).

This technique tests the general synchronization of the fasciae, especially the thoracic and cervicocranial fasciae. Mild suboccipital traction affects all the posterior fasciae.

In the normal situation, the hands should sense a full, free, and rhythmic movement. If problems are present, the movement will be asynchronous and will tend to prefer certain directions over others.

7-13 Anteroposterior Listening Test

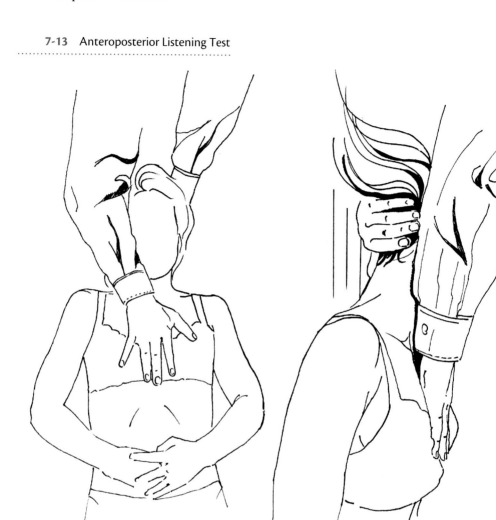

Effects of stress on listening

In certain highly stressed individuals, tissue motility will be perturbed, with movement slowed down and reduced in amplitude. What is felt will be a lack of freedom in the floating of the tissues, as if they were uncertain in which direction they should be moving. In addition, there will be a feeling of retraction and the hand will feel like it wants to clench. This can be felt anywhere, but is most evident around the cranium and in the thorax, most commonly over the sternum.

Special areas

Certain parts of the body are more vulnerable and retain particularly long-lasting impressions when subject to any kind of injury. The fasciae in these areas could be said to have a particularly long-term memory. Placing the hands over these areas is often sufficient to detect fascial tensions that are secondary to very ancient insults.

These areas are concentrated over the cranium, the cervical vertebrae, the upper thoracic vertebrae, the sternum, the coccyx, and the epigastrium, as well as in scar tissue and at original points of impact.

Cranium and cervical vertebrae

The region of the cranium and cervical spine represents an important crossroads for nerves and blood vessels. It is also highly mobile, which serves a functional role, but is also important in adaptation and compensation mechanisms. The region of the upper cervical vertebrae and the base of the skull is a focus for a multitude of constraints, and is in a constant state of readjustment in order to insure optimal functioning at the higher information processing and command centers.

In the event of severe trauma, it is the cervical vertebrae and the occipitocervical junction which represent the ultimate point at which damage can be attenuated. Therefore, it is not surprising that fascial tension and restricted mobility is not uncommon in this region—it is not going too far to say that it is rare not to find some kind of problem here. The most common kinds of tension to leave their mark here are those related to childbirth.

A fairly common phenomenon is lateral translation of the cervical vertebrae with compensation between the atlas and the occiput. This is usually the result of a traffic accident or some other kind of shock from the side. More often than not, the patient has completely forgotten the original event, but the tissues have not.

Upper thoracic vertebrae

The upper thoracic vertebrae support the cervical vertebrae and are often distorted as a result of overlying distortion. For example, after a rabbit punch, it is often this region which is obliged to absorb much of the excess energy and which, as a result, becomes pathological. One of the most dangerous types of shock is that associated with a fall flat on the back, especially when the person is still a child. Such a shock sets up a serious chain of events, including respiratory spasm, which can lead to anxiety and even panic attacks.

Such an injury, together with its associated stress, will leave its mark on the tissues. When we put our hand on this area, we will feel marked rigidity and tension in the tissues, as if the skin were too tightly stretched. It usually suffices to simply ask the patient if anything happened to learn about the injury, because it will have left an unforgettable impression.

Moreover, as previously discussed, the upper thoracic region is a very important fascial meeting point which is constantly working. As a result of shocks, stress, and tension, this region is subject to an ever-increasing number of restrictions of steadily mounting severity, ultimately resulting in changes in local static properties. The back begins to arch and the shoulders slide forward—leading to the rather telling expression, "I'm carrying the whole world on my shoulders!"

Sternum

This is a common site for tension secondary to repeated, uncompensated stress.

A listening test here may show the tissues to be tense and fixed, with a tendency to retract towards the center. This can leave the impression that the hand is growing hollow while the sternum is retracting in a posterior direction. In victims of motor vehicle accidents, the seat belt can often leave a restriction, which is easy to detect in a listening test in the form of an oblique pulling of the hand, crossing the upper thorax.

Coccyx

In the same way as a fall flat on the back leaves a lasting impression, anyone who has ever fallen on their coccyx is unlikely to forget it. If there is an instance where the expression "seeing stars" is applicable, it is when this region is hurt. Apart from any local damage, a fall on the coccyx is often associated with shocks in the abdomen and thorax, which can travel all the way up to the cranium. After such an injury, it is not uncommon to develop painful tension in one of the organs, and even a prolapse can result.

As a result of this shock, the coccyx is usually injured in flexion and side-bending. Local palpation can detect the effects of such a shock many years later, even if it has become silent. We can say that the impression is there for life.

Epigastrium

Many people somatize stress to the epigastrium—an idea embodied in the expression about having "butterflies in one's stomach." Such stress will stimulate the solar plexus, which will in turn have repercussions throughout the abdominal region.

Listening in such a region will give the impression of a hard, overly tense area, depression of which is resisted and causes pain. Palpation gives an impression of a hard ball being under the hand. The organs are immobile and distended. Just the fact of placing the hand induces very pronounced aortic pulsation, which can be particularly worrying for the patient.

Scars

Not all scars lead to loss of function, but, as we have seen, it is not uncommon. They therefore must be tested systematically because, when they become disruptive, they constitute the primary cause of mechanical or physiological impairment. A listening test can easily reveal the direction of any tension being induced by a restrictive scar.

Impact points

When the body experiences a shock, it must be absorbed in some way in order to avoid damage to fragile internal structures. The energy of a direct impact like a punch is first attenuated by the skin, the fasciae, and the adipose cushion. When a blow strikes a relatively poorly protected region where the shock absorbing capacity of the tissues is limited, such as the tibia or skull, the effect on the underlying fasciae is all the more pronounced. This can create restrictions which correspond to the points of departure of a pathological lesion or restriction. Such 'traces' of shock impact points must be sought assiduously because they are often key to the success of our treatment strategy.

Shocks to the cranium, especially those to the posterolateral part, can cause changes in the connective tissue which lead to a descending chain reaction of damage, transmitted through successive structures from the area of occipitocervical junction through the cervical vertebrae, the cervicothoracic junction, and the shoulder.

In a listening test, the most common observation is point-like restriction. Serious shocks, such as those incurred in traffic accidents or through a fall onto the wrist, can overwhelm the shock-absorbing capacity of the soft tissues and must therefore be dealt with by stronger structures, namely, the bone-periosteum complex. Bone has a certain degree of plasticity and is constructed in such a way as to absorb shocks. However, strong shocks will nevertheless leave an impression on bone tissue and can trigger a pathological process.

Relevant here is a recent case history of a patient who had been involved in a head-on collision in his car. The patient had been gripping the steering wheel and most of the energy was transmitted to his left radius. A listening test indicated that the bone was compressed to a certain extent, and that the fibers of the tissue intercalated with one another. In fact, the bone had almost broken.

Palpation and Mobility Tests

PALPATION

Listening tests are purely passive and are performed using the entire surface of the hand. By contrast, palpation is performed with the digital pad at the tips of the fingers and involves the exertion of varying degrees of pressure, depending on the area to be reached.

Before continuing, here we will make a short digression. Before touching the patient, it is vital to make a visual assessment of the area to be tested; the information so obtained can be extremely useful. Things to look for are the color and condition of the skin, including whether it is thick or thin, and whether any spots, blemishes, or lumps are present. For example, a slight curving of the linea alba off to the side indicates some kind of problem in the area corresponding to the direction of the curve. Remember that the skin, through the intermediary of the Heine cylinders discussed in Chapter 3, can reveal what is happening in the deeper tissues.

The purpose of palpation is to detect any change which might have occurred in a tissue. Such changes may be structural or the foci of pain.

Structural changes

Structural changes will be observed first in the skin and then in the underlying fasciae, according to a progression from the outermost layer to the interior.

In the skin

Normal skin is flexible, regular, and elastic. Abnormal skin may be:

- indurated

- infiltrated
- edematous

Moreover, abnormal skin may have lost some or all of its natural elasticity. Sometimes, it will be impossible to create a skin fold and, in other cases, the fold will persist for a relatively long time, indicating modification of the cross-linking bonds.

In the underlying fasciae

The fasciae immediately below the skin should be thought of as flexible sheets which have, nevertheless, a certain degree of firmness. Different fasciae have different degrees of firmness, from the most easily depressible regions, like the anterior neck, to areas where the fasciae must be particularly strong, like insertion points, ligaments, and some of the mesenteries.

As a general rule, a healthy fascia may or may not have ridges, and is composed of parallel bands all aligned in the same direction. Distortion of its structure will modify its viscoelastic properties and change the way it feels on palpation. A loss of elasticity will translate as increased resistance to palpation—the fascia will feel abnormally tight, and more force will be required to penetrate it.

Changes to collagen fibers in the fascia will manifest in a variety of ways:

- Some bands of fascia will be noticeably tighter than neighboring structures. Sometimes, these will have a sharply-defined edge, oriented obliquely or at a right angle to the general direction of the fibers. These bands are indicative of abnormal influences and they are directed towards the focus of the problem. They are easy to palpate and, on dissection, are seen to be due to relatively dense bundles of fibers which have a particularly pearly sheen.
- There will be abnormally tense bands of fascia twisting around a longitudinal axis parallel to the general direction of the fibers—usually longer than the oblique of perpendicular bands.
- Certain fasciae, like the fascia lata, are naturally ridged: under the influence of excessive tension, the ridges have a tendency to become more pronounced, analogous to what happens when a curtain is drawn.
- In other circumstances, within a fascial band or a normal fascia, small nodules can be felt. Most of these are oval in shape and can vary in size from that of a grain of rice to that of an olive stone; other, rounder nodules can vary in size from that of a grain of sand to one of sea salt. The oval-shaped nodules are usually found in the membranes which separate muscles; the rounder ones can occur anywhere. All these nodules are hard, approaching the hardness of bone tissue.
- Finally, palpation may reveal areas that are extremely indurated or even calcified. These can extend for a matter of a few millimeters to as far as two centimeters. Such indurated areas are most commonly found around the shoulder, the elbow, the deep vertebral ligaments, and the plantar aponeurosis.

These areas have such a hard texture because what is happening is that soft tissue is in the process of being converted into bone. In response to stress which is too great, the fascia, ligament, or muscle is starting to calcify. This phenomenon which leads to the ossification of soft tissue has been extensively studied by Stevenson et al., who concluded that it is the bone-producing protein osteogenin that makes it possible to convert muscle tissue into bone.

As will be discussed later, this process is not always—happily for us—irreversible.

Pain

It is said that pain is often misleading, and that it should be treated with caution in light of both the amount of variability among patients, and the fact that it can mask underlying problems. Nevertheless, when taken into account with the appropriate precautions, it can be a very useful indicator.

Mild pressure exerted on a fascia should not cause pain. However, if it is damaged, its sensitivity can be markedly enhanced and it can become frankly painful, especially in the vicinity of the above-mentioned bands and nodules. This can mean that the patient can barely stand even very light palpation in calcified fasciae or around certain compromised ligaments. Extremely acute pain—such as that following a burn—can be triggered by even a very light touch.

Pain is associated with the release of certain prostaglandins. Aspirin and other pain killers block prostaglandin synthesis and thereby prevent the effects of this critical group of substances, the function of which is to sound the alarm that tissue damage has occurred or is occurring.

Effective treatment always results in a major reduction in the number of painful foci, and sometimes in their complete disappearance. Apart from the immediate benefit in terms of the actual pain itself, this has another, perhaps less obvious advantage, in that it helps to convince the patient of the validity of the approach. After all, he or she only came to see you because of "a pain there." So, although pain may represent no more than the tip of the iceberg, it is nevertheless one of the factors that come together to constitute the osteopathic lesion.

MOBILITY TESTS

Mobility tests follow on naturally from palpation—they are closely associated.

Purpose of mobility tests

The purpose of this type of test is to detect any impairment of mobility, be it in the skin, a ligament, an internal structure, or a joint. It is a follow-up modality to confirm the findings of a listening test.

Since mobility testing is relevant to all parts of the body, it requires a very profound understanding of anatomy. The more advanced our understanding of the anatomical structures being palpated, the higher will be the resolution of our

mobility testing, and, as a result, the more effective the treatment strategy.
There are two different types of mobility tests:

- long lever tests
- local tests

Long lever tests

Long lever tests, sometimes referred to as sectional tests, are performed on segments or more extensive areas. Restriction in a particular joint or area may be due to a purely local cause, but it may also be derived from fascial tension elsewhere which is creating a long lesional chain.

These are the classic tests that involve the movement and quality of a general area: plantar flexion, dorsal flexion, anterior flexion of the head or the trunk, etc. They are easy to perform, although it is not so easy for beginners to pin down at the outset whether the restriction is purely local or part of a long fascial lever. With some practice, however, it is easy to tell the difference. It is important to make this distinction because the required corrective action depends not only on the character of the restriction, but also on the area under consideration.

Unfortunately, these long lever tests are often ignored or performed improperly. Nevertheless, it is this kind of test which gives the patient an objective demonstration of the improvement mediated by the treatment in the form of enhanced mobility, an enhancement which is often accompanied by a reduction in the level of pain.

Local tests

A local test is a specific test designed to establish an accurate diagnosis of the pathological focus. It defines the nature of the restriction, its location, and its depth. It naturally follows on from listening tests and palpation, and is used to confirm or exclude the possibilities already raised. In the end, it leads directly to the treatment, so the more effective the execution of the test, the more suitable and effective the strategy eventually adopted is likely to be. Of course, all this assumes that the practitioner has extensive experience in palpation and an intimate and accurate knowledge of anatomical topography.

We will discuss local tests from the outside in, starting at the surface and going down from there through the deeper tissues, from the skin through the superficial and deep fasciae to the internal organs.

Skin

The bottommost layer of the skin is attached to the superficial fascia. As previously discussed, a problem in the deep tissues can have effects at the skin, whether it be changes in skin structure or an actual lesional chain involving both superficial and deeper elements. Depending on the size of the area, the method involves using either the pad at the tips of two or three fingers or the entire hand to gently manipulate the skin in all directions. In simple terms, all one is doing is sliding one plane of tissues over another.

In the normal situation, the mobility of the skin should be similar in all directions, while if there is any restriction present, the mobility of the skin in that direction will be reduced or missing altogether, thus giving an immediate indication of the location of the restriction and its direction. By increasing the pressure, one can reach deeper tissues and test different planes.

Peripheral fasciae

We are not going to try to describe all the various tests for all the fasciae—modalities are more or less the same for all segments. However, we will go over some of the most common tests and some of those which can be key for our treatment strategies.

▶ LOWER LIMB

Plantar aponeurosis. With the patient lying prone, flex the knee so that plantar aspect of the foot is facing upwards and exert pressure on the plantar aponeurosis. Soon, you will feel a cord under your fingers. As you increase the pressure, the pain level will rise until it can no longer be tolerated.

Next, hook the pad of your last three or four fingers around the internal edge of the ligament and pull it towards the outside. If there is a restriction present, the movement will soon be restricted and the patient will experience pain (Fig. 7-14).

Fig. 7-14 Plantar Aponeurosis Test

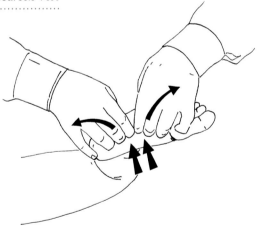

Anteromedial fascia of the leg. This fascia lies directly over the tibia. With the patient supine, slide the tips of two or three fingers along the fascia from the ankle to the knee (Fig. 7-15). If there are any restrictions, you will encounter an edematous patch of skin which will block the passage of your finger. Focusing here, try to move the skin and the underlying fascia. This movement will be resisted and may cause pain—the fascia seems to be stuck to the periosteum. Sometimes, you will observe a small fascial band which will block the advance of your finger; in the chapter on treatment, we will discuss why it is important to investigate this kind of restriction.

Fig. 7-15 Testing the Anteromedial Fascia of the Leg

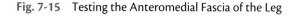
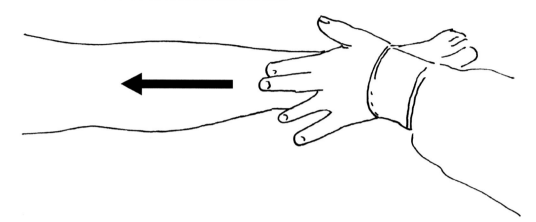

Anterolateral and posterolateral compartments of the leg. This test involves the planes of juxtaposition of the muscular fasciae and the tibia. With the patient supine, the knee is bent and the foot placed flat on the table. With the tips of both thumbs, moving from the ankle towards the knee, feel the anterolateral compartment; the posterior muscular compartment is evaluated with the finger tips (Figs. 7-16 & 7-17). If there are any restrictions, it will be difficult to reach the deeper tissues with the fingers and the patient will feel pain if you try. This test can be very useful for the sequelae of sciatica, a fracture, sprained ankle, or refractory pain in the calf.

Fig. 7-16 Testing the Posteromedial Compartment of the Leg

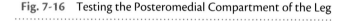
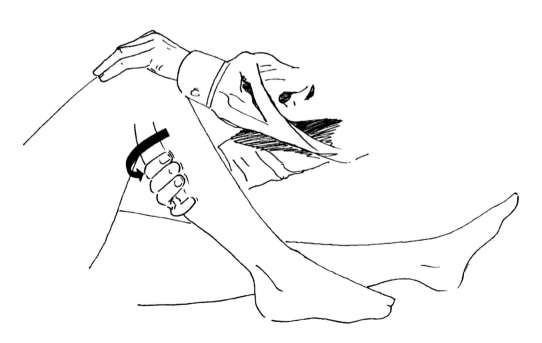

Fig. 7-17   Testing the Anterolateral Compartment of the Leg

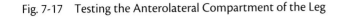

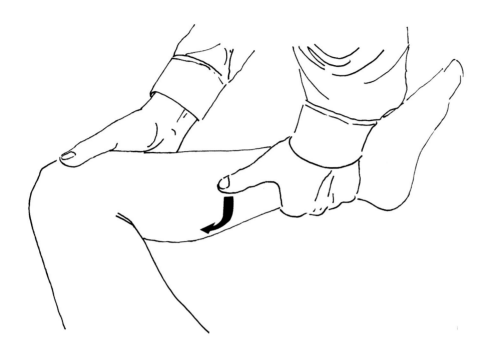

Sciatic nerve fascia. Throughout its length, the sciatic nerve is invested by a kind of fascial protection. In the normal situation, the sciatic nerve cannot be felt in palpation but this can change in the event of pathology.

With the patient prone, the practitioner takes up a position to the side of the patient.

Begin palpation at the gluteal fold. Remember that the sciatic nerve runs down the length of the thigh, along the cleavage plane between the biceps femoris on one side and the semimembranosus and semitendinosus muscles on the other. Find this cleavage plane and steadily penetrate deeper and deeper with the finger tips, and try to manipulate the deep planes in the longitudinal and transverse directions (Fig. 7-18).

Continue on down through the popliteal fossa to the Achilles tendon, passing between the two gemellus muscles. At this level, it is sometimes useful to place the knee in mild flexion (Fig. 7-19).

In patients with sciatic pathology, it will be difficult to move the deep planes and any attempt to do so will induce pain. As a general rule, restrictions tend to occur in the upper part of the thigh and in the middle part of the calf. Most commonly, the focus of the restriction consists of an area extending over several centimeters. However, sometimes the focus of the restriction will be relatively short and located at the junction between the top one-third and the bottom two-thirds of the thigh.

Fig. 7-18   Sciatic Nerve Fascia Test (Proximal)

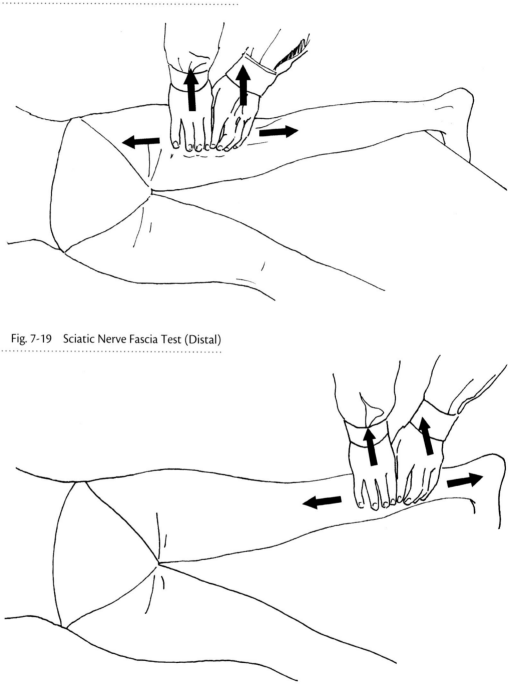

Fig. 7-19   Sciatic Nerve Fascia Test (Distal)

► BACK

Gluteal and vertebral muscles. With the patient prone, the practitioner stands to one side. The fingertips are used to feel the upper insertion planes of the gluteal muscles under the iliac crest (Fig. 7-20). In this region, it is common to find extremely tense, painful fascial bands which are seriously disturbing the mechanics of the pelvis.

Continue to use the finger tips to feel back along the vertebral muscles as far up as the cervicothoracic region, possibly carrying on up to the occipitocervical junction (Fig. 7-21). If one goes deep enough, you will fairly often encounter bundles of fibers which roll below the fingers. These bundles can be as thick as a finger.

A tense area may be found starting at the inferior lumbar level and extending upwards without interruption to fairly high in the thoracics. It is worth following such a tense area upwards because often its termination point corresponds to some kind of thoracic restriction which is causally related to that of the lumbar region.

At the superior thoracic level, you may encounter obliquely aligned bands of fascia which are associated with the medial muscular attachment points of the scapula and the posterior and superior serratus muscles. At this point, there is a belt which corresponds to where fibers running in different directions cross over one another.

Fig. 7-20   Testing the Gluteal Fasciae   **Fig. 7-21**   Testing the Fasciae of the Paravertebral Muscles

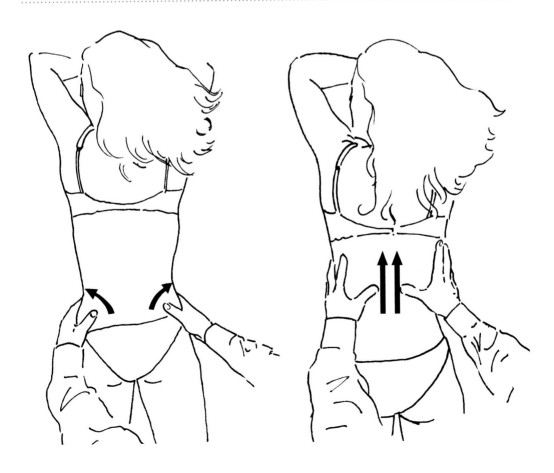

Scapula. With the patient prone, the practitioner stands to the side and places their hands flat over the two scapulas. Move them in all directions to test how easily the underlying planes of tissue slide over one another (*Fig. 7-22*).

Next, specifically test the areas above and below the spine of the scapula with the finger tips. Above the spine, you will find areas of painful tension located between the muscle fibers and oriented horizontally. Below the spine, the areas of tension will be obliquely aligned in the direction of the shoulder, with the most revealing points concentrated around the lateral, superior edge of the scapula. These are the areas where the problems lie in the majority of patients with shoulder problems.

Fig. 7-22 Scapular Test

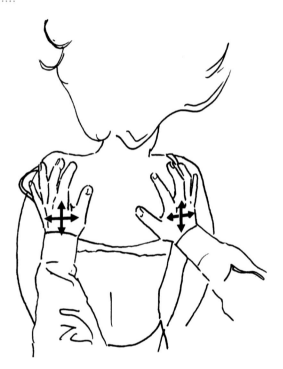

▶ ANTERIOR TRUNK

We will focus on two particularly active areas, the sternum and the clavicle.

Sternum. With the patient supine the practitioner stands to the side and places one hand completely flat on the sternum as for a listening test. When well-positioned over the sternum, move it in all directions. Over the sternum, the fascia is in direct contact with the bone, as is the case over the tibia. To make things easier, you can use both hands by crossing them, with the base of one on the sternal notch, and that of the other over the xiphoid process (*Fig. 7-23*).

Slide your finger tips along the sternum. If there is a restriction present, your passage will be blocked by a horizontally oriented fibrous barrier. Foci of restrictions—often hyper-acute—will be encountered around the median line and in the cartilaginous parts of the sternum.

The sternum is a very hard-working area, and is active in all movements affecting the thorax. Fascial problems here are common. Moreover, as previously noted, this region is particularly susceptible to all types of stress-related problems.

Clavicle. The clavicle is a meeting point for different fascial elements as well as being a consistently hard-working region. It can cause problems in the overlying structures and also, because of its underlying attachments, in the brachial plexus and the subclavian artery. The test is mainly relevant to subclavian structures, that is, the clavipectoral fascia and the conoid, trapezoid, and acromioclavicular ligaments.

Fig. 7-23 Sternum Test

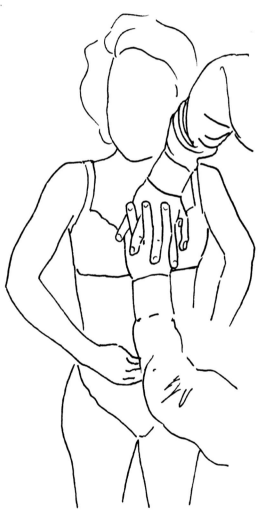

The test is done with the patient supine and the practitioner standing to the side, with their thumb and index finger on either side of the clavicle. Gradually feel around the clavicle in order to reach the underlying soft tissues (Fig. 7-24). If the tissues in this area completely relax, the two fingers will be able to meet on the inferior side of the bone. If some kind of tension is present, penetration is inhibited and the patient soon feels pain.

To make things easier, you can have the patient raise the contralateral arm; better still, position the patient on their side, which will relax them most effectively. If the tension is acute, this last position is more suitable for palpation.

Fig. 7-24   Clavicular Fasciae Test

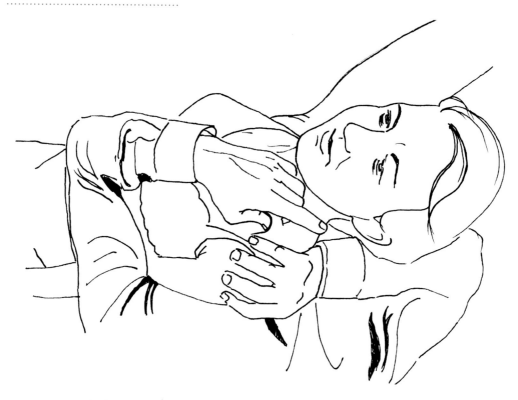

▶ NECK

Here, we will just cover a test for the cartilaginous tissue and for the pharyngobasilar fascia.

This is a very important region in the regulation of the pharynx, the larynx, and the thyroid gland. As was described in the anatomy chapter, this zone articulates with the cervical vertebrae. The hyoid bone is an important shock absorber and dissipator of tensions which are transmitted via the central axis and from other sources.

The hyoid bone and thyroid cartilage are mechanically linked in the process of voice production, with the cartilage attached to the hyoid bone to provide play in the arytenoid cartilage and thereby make the vocal cords vibrate. Remember that the vocal cords vibrate at about 20,000 Hertz (rising to 36,000 in the case of the highest soprano voices). Obviously, even the mildest disruption in this region can have serious consequences for the voice, among other physiological functions.

General test for the neck. With the patient supine, the practitioner stands to the side and places their cephalad hand on the patient's forehead. Three fingers of the other hand are placed along the contralateral side of the visceral axis of the neck, while the thumb is placed on the ipsilateral side.

First, turn the head towards the left and, at the same time, exert some traction towards the right using the finger tips (Fig. 7-25). Then turn the head towards the right while pushing gently with the thumb towards the left. For greater specificity, one can take the axis of the neck between thumb and index finger and test segment by segment.

If there are any restrictions, the mobility of the neck will be reduced and the manipulations may induce acute pain. When performing this test, a reflex cough is a very common response, especially when the fixed side is mobilized at the thyroid-cricoid level.

Fig. 7-25   General Neck Test

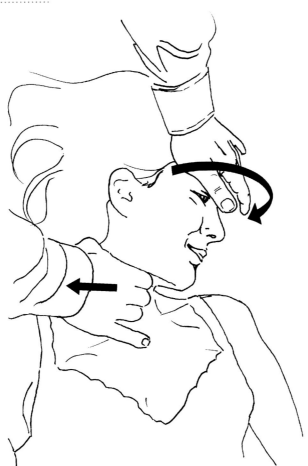

It is not unusual to observe the following phenomena when performing this general test:

- A rubbing noise can be heard, which can be very loud in certain cases. Sometimes this noise is perfectly normal; what is not normal is if it is associated with pain, usually retropharyngeal, and projected onto the cervical vertebrae.
- Acute pain can be felt, induced by stretching at the level of one of the cervical vertebrae. This is often associated with symptoms at the same spot reported by the patient.

It is important not to forget that the visceral axis of the neck is linked to the anterior processes of the transverse fasciae by the fibrous tract that has an antero-posterior orientation.

Hyoid bone. Palpating the hyoid bone can provide information about a number of different structures, including the superficial and middle cervical fasciae, and the pharyngobasilar fascia. Palpating it will also let us better appreciate its relationship with the styloid process of the temporal bone via the Riolan bouquet and its relationship with the scapula via the omohyoid muscle.

The hyoid bone is a U-shaped fibrocartilaginous structure and it is this shape which makes human speech possible; the equivalent in animals is different, having a far more open structure. However, there is significant normal anatomical variation in the shape of this structure. In many individuals, usually women, the hyoid bone is relatively closed, like a tuning fork, whereas in many others, more commonly men, it is often open, like a pair of antlers.

The test is done with the patient supine and the practitioner on the side, with the sides of the hyoid bone placed between the thumb and index finger of their caudal hand. The bone is displaced to the right and the left, and then anteriorly and posteriorly (Fig. 7-26). It is then tilted to the side by one finger on its lower part and the opposite finger on its upper part. One side will often be found to be higher than the other (usually the left-hand side), but, as long as the tension remains moderate, this can be considered as a normal variation.

The next step is to palpate the entire anterior aspect of the throat. This is done by taking the thyroid cartilage between thumb and index finger of one hand and the hyoid bone in the other. Then move the hyoid bone back and forth with respect to the thyroid cartilage (Fig. 7-27).

Hyoid-cricoid test. This is another important subhyoid cartilage that should be tested. The patient remains supine and the hyoid-cricoid cartilage is taken between the thumb and index finger. Each structure is moved with respect to the other to test its flexibility and the presence of any restrictions.

▶ CRANIUM

Mobility testing around the skull involves manipulating the scalp with respect to the underlying bone tissue. In the normal situation, the skin slides over the bone without either tension or pain. Obviously, the skin over the forehead and the base of the skull is more mobile than elsewhere.

If there are any foci of restriction (secondary to the kind of shock we have already discussed), a variety of phenomena can be observed:

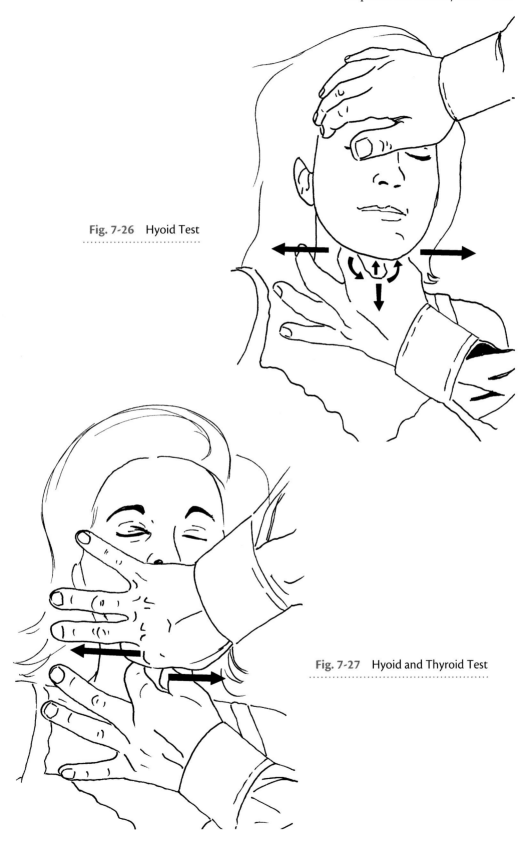

Fig. 7-26   Hyoid Test

Fig. 7-27   Hyoid and Thyroid Test

- A very tense, easily isolated band of fascial tissue may be felt, sometimes feeling like a small thread, a few centimeters in length. This type of tension is most common in the parietotemporal region.
- An edematous, infiltrated area with a diameter of the order of two centimeters may be felt. The middle of this area is often depressed, corresponding to the focus of the restriction affecting the periosteum. Such zones are very difficult to move and are often associated with pain like that due to a sting by an insect (which can be acute).
- A hollow patch over the bone may be found. This is encountered at the suture sites and over the sutural bones. The finger will feel a depressed area, as if the fascia is being sucked down towards the interior. In these areas too, attempts to displace the tissue will induce pain.

Abdomen

We do not intend to exhaustively cover all the tests for the viscera, but we would emphasize the importance of palpation and mobility testing in the abdomen. If there is one region of the body in which osteopathy is purely applied anatomy, it is this one. For correct diagnosis and effective treatment strategies, when it comes to pappation, it is essential to be completely familiar with the topographic anatomy of the region and with all its characteristics.

Listening tests can be of enormous utility in the diagnostic process, but they can never be enough on their own. Both palpation and mobility testing must be performed as well. Apart from the fact that palpation reveals areas which are sensitive or which contain points of restriction, the technique is also essential for understanding the exact status of an area which has been detected as abnormal in a listening test.

It is obvious that if a practitioner detects irregular bumps, areas of induration, or deformations under their fingers, caution should be the watchword and the patient should be referred to the appropriate specialist. Such morphological changes can only be detected through careful palpation by an experienced practitioner.

The problems which arise with the abdomen are related to the depth of the tissues to be palpated, and the fact that many other structures may lie between the surface and the element of interest. This complicates the process of differential diagnosis. Nevertheless, with a combination of practice and intimate knowledge of the local anatomy, such diagnosis is often possible.

Palpation, as has already been emphasized, must be as accurate as possible. Therefore, depending on the structure of interest, it must sometimes be deep, and also, despite intervening structures, it must concern the relevant area itself, rather than some projection of it. If we are patient and look carefully for the most appropriate route of access, the fasciae almost always let us through; thus, without too much difficulty, we can manage to palpate even a mesenteric artery, the suspensory muscle of the duodenum, or a kidney via the anterior approach.

Abdominal palpation should be immediately followed by a mobility test on the organ, mesentery, or ligament in question. Mobility varies enormously between different segments: for example, while the intestines are extremely mobile, the liver and the ligaments are much less so, and it is practically impossible to significantly displace the suspensory muscle of the duodenum or a mesenteric artery. However, it should never be forgotten that all tissues have some degree of elasticity—it is this that one is testing when one is focused on a region or structure with very limited mobility.

Abdominal palpation and mobility testing can be unpleasant for the patient, even painful. But acute pain should put the practitioner on guard. Unlike the case of the peripheral fasciae, where almost intolerable pain can occur in the absence of any major health problem, acute pain in the abdomen may well indicate serious pathology and should be treated accordingly.

Scars and adhesions

▶ SCARS

As previously discussed, foreign material can be trapped in scar tissue and this can disturb a variety of physiological and biological processes. In addition, scars can trigger adhesions which will inevitably change the viscoelastic properties of the local tissues and thereby lead to loss of function. Therefore, all scars must be systematically investigated.

Apart from palpating the superficial tissue and the surface of the scar, it is also important to test the mobility of the underlying scar tissue. Using the tips of one or two fingers, manipulate the entire area of scar tissue in all directions, making sure to penetrate deep enough; the exact depth will depend on the location of the scar. If there are any adhesions, there will be a clear blockage offering more or less resistance to the displacement of the tissue. In most cases, the adhesion follows one specific axis.

▶ ADHESIONS

Adhesions secondary to infection or inflammation (as opposed to scarring) tend to be less 'visible' and can only be detected by palpation and mobility testing. As a general rule, such adhesions are located in the viscera, the true pelvis, the abdomen, and the thorax. Post mortem dissection often reveals the presence of fibrous bridges between the pleura and the lungs; the problem here is that this tissue is impossible to reach directly.

SPECIAL CASES

We will consider the tests for certain ligaments separately because they correspond to very common problems which represent a significant proportion of osteopathic practice, and respond well to osteopathic treatment.

These ligaments are the:

- iliolumbar
- sacrotuberous and sacrospinous
- anterior longitudinal
- cervicopleural

Iliolumbar ligaments

We will describe the test for the right iliolumbar ligament. The patient should be standing, with their legs slightly apart. The practitioner stands behind the patient and is in contact with them. Your left arm is under the patient's left arm, encircling the lower part of the patient's chest. Slide your right thumb along the descending part of the iliac crest, moving downwards and forwards to arrive at the space between L4 and L5, where you will encounter the iliolumbar ligament.

In some patients, the ligament will be completely relaxed and difficult to feel. In most however, it will be tense, easily isolated, and slightly sensitive. Its diameter is similar to that of a pencil. In a third group of patients, it is so tense that it feels calcified, and it is difficult to displace and extremely sensitive.

In order to make palpation easier, you can perform a leftward translation of the pelvis at the same time as inclining the trunk to the right, and, if necessary, rotating the patient to the right as well (Fig. 7-28). Support the patient on your left arm so that he or she remains completely relaxed.

This test for this ligament is only effective and meaningful if the patient is standing upright. With the patient supine, the result is of little relevance because the static properties of this ligament mean that, unless it is supporting some weight, it is not working and is therefore difficult to test.

Dissection reveals that the iliolumbar ligament is actually a circular structure, similar in size to a pencil. It has a particularly pearly sheen, bearing witness to the changes in connective tissue structure induced by extremely heavy work.

Sacrotuberous and sacrospinous ligaments

Here, we will just mention some important relevant points. First, the patient should be prone when palpating for these ligaments, which are subject to huge tensions, so that sometimes they feel positively indurated. The sacrospinous ligament is more difficult to detect because it lies below a major mass of muscle tissue. When palpating these, always bear in mind their relationship with the piriformis muscle and the sciatic nerve. Finally, do not forget that the sciatic ligaments are related to the pelvic region

Anterior longitudinal ligament

It is sometimes worth testing this ligament in patients with lumbosacral problems. To do so, have the patient lie supine, with their knees bent, and stand to the side. Place the finger tips of both hands on the lower part of the linea alba. Gradually and gently, descend until you come into contact with the bone. This may take some time and it does require finesse. Perform a longitudinal stretching manipulation while spreading the fingers of each hand in opposite directions. Then, very gently, perform a transverse stretching manipulation (Fig. 7-29).

Fig. 7-28 Iliolumbar Ligament Test

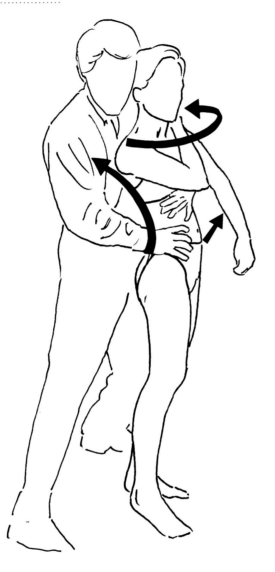

Palpation of this ligament can sometimes induce acute pain, which spreads to the lumbosacral region or even as far as one of the nerve roots. It is evident that this test is only possible with thinner patients whose abdomen can be depressed without too much difficulty. It is not worth attempting to perform in a plethoric patient. It is generally easier in women.

It is almost not worth specifying that this palpation must terminate at the aortic bifurcation.

Cervicopleural ligaments

Three in number, these ligaments attach the cervicothoracic diaphragm to the first rib and the cervical vertebrae. They are, going anteriorly from the back, the:

Fig. 7-29   Anterior Longitudinal Ligament Test

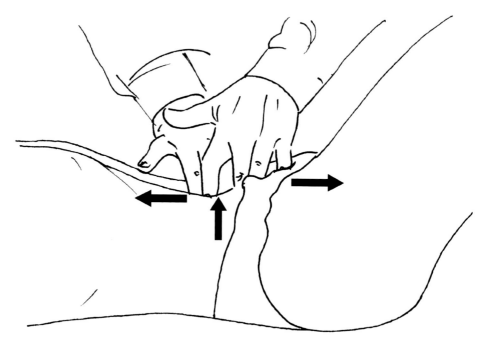

- costopleural ligament
- transverse cupular ligament
- pleurovertebral ligament

In the normal situation, these ligaments are very difficult to isolate, but, if there is significant tension, they can be easily felt. This is done with the patient supine and the practitioner behind their head. We will describe the test done on the right side.

In order to make palpation easier, slightly raise the patient's head and side-bend it to the right, with your right thumb in front of the trapezius muscle up to the level of T1, that is, of the costopleural ligament. After this has been clearly felt, move your thumb anteriorly by drawing an arc of a circle in a forward direction to try and isolate first the transverse cupulare ligament, and then the pleurovertebral ligament (Fig. 7-30).

This palpation can be performed with the patient sitting, but this will make it more difficult because of other fascial tensions which will be superimposed.

Remember that the cervicothoracic ganglion is located close to the costopleural ligament, and that the ligament itself splits into two branches before it terminates. The T1 root passes through these two branches.

TIMING OF TESTS

Once an area has been tested—wherever it is in the body—a certain schedule should be followed in order to maximize the amount of information gathered:

Fig. 7-30 Cervico-Pleural Ligament Test

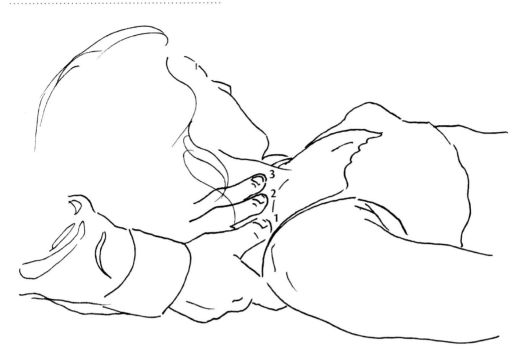

- First of all, learn how to inspect the area visually. As previously mentioned, this can be highly instructive.
- Next, perform a motility test, which achieves two ends, in that it both reassures the patient and permits you to initiate the contact with their tissues.
- Then perform palpation and mobility tests.

We reiterate that it is dangerous to depend on any single parameter. In osteopathy, the diagnostic procedure is one of convergence based on accumulating as much information as possible—including clinical findings, radiological images, and the results of medical, listening, and mobility tests—in order to identify the etiology of the patient's problem with as small a margin of error as possible.

8

Treating the Fasciae

Objectives of Treatment

Any insult, whatever its nature, will have some kind of effect on tissue structure. The injured tissue will change texture to become more granular, edematous, or indurated with a concomitant increase in the sensitivity of the local muscles and fascial elements. These changes, through biochemical and physical phenomena, will cause loss of fascial function which will, in turn, induce changes in the physiological behavior of parts of the body or organs.

Bednar et al. have documented degenerative changes in fasciae due to the separation of bundles of collagen fibers with the concomitant formation of myxoid tissue, which is heavily infiltrated by lymphocytes and plasma cells. Vascular proliferation is associated in certain patients with abnormal capillaries without any external basement membrane, and in others with the presence of tiny foci of calcification.

As previously discussed, if the insult is extreme or sustained for too long a time, exchange processes between the ground substance and cells will be affected. This can cause intracellular regulatory problems which can become chronic and cause morbidity.

One of the major etiologies of the loss of fascial function is trauma. Following any serious accident, one must consider the effects on the fasciae of all parts of the body. Changes in the tissues may be immediate or may only appear in the hours or days following the traumatic event. Treatment of such injuries should begin as soon as possible, preferably with fascial techniques.

Changes within connective tissue will have effects on both the sensory and sympathetic nervous systems. This will lead to perturbation of afferent impulses which will, in turn, cause spinal facilitation, thereby creating a vicious cycle. Facilitation of sympathetic transmission will disrupt a variety of processes, including glandular function, secretory processes, vasomotor activity, and organ function.

Increased sympathetic tonus can, frankly, be dangerous. In the normal situation, the sympathetic nervous system plays a very important role in the protective and adaptive adjustments made to the internal milieu in response to changes in the outside environment, muscular effort, emotional stress, and so forth. Notably, it inhibits the activity of internal organs, which are not directly involved in the response to such situations, and reduces the amount of blood flowing to these organs and to the skin, redirecting it to striated muscle tissue. These periods are usually relatively brief and are followed by a period of respite and rest. Persistent sympathicotonia, however, will lead to reduced blood flow and secretory activity, as well as sphincteral spasm, which will eventually result in tissue damage and loss of function in the part of the organs concerned.

It should be noted that clinical symptoms may evolve over time. Hyperhydrosis can turn into hypohydrosis, and angiospasm can give way to vasomotor atony with stasis, inflammation, and edema. In other words, a chronic state begins to produce degenerative changes. Sympathicotonia which may be obvious at the beginning cannot remain so and tends to become masked in some way.

In the endocrine system, prolonged sympathicotonia will affect the responses of tissues to circulating hormones. Similarly, it can lead to local relative ischemia in the endocrine glands themselves that is likely to have far-reaching effects. These can occur in tissues distant from the actual gland that is compromised or the area which is facilitated.

The processes which are triggered in the facilitated segment mean that, once established, facilitation can persist long after the disappearance of the stimulus which originally induced the response. This is the meaning of facilitation.

Taking these various pieces of information together, it becomes evident that damage to connective tissue can induce—in the shorter or longer term—a lesional process which subsequently becomes self-perpetuating through the action of the nervous system. The role of the nervous system in this process is to create a state of facilitation, thereby generating a vicious cycle which, if it is not broken, will result in degenerative processes and physiological disturbance at some point in the more or less distant future.

The goal of the osteopathic approach is therefore to break this cycle by correcting spasm, tension, and tissular irritation, as well as reversing the sympathicotonia, so that the functionality of the fasciae can be restored in full.

Releasing tissues and correcting posture are of primordial importance in the maintenance of blood flow. As long as the hemodynamic picture is not disturbed, tissue exchange processes will occur completely normally. The tissues will all be adequately supplied with all the substances that they need for normal functioning (hormones, nutrients, etc.), and the waste products of metabolic processes will be efficiently removed, thereby avoiding local stasis, which can cause serious problems. When the nervous system is free of problems, it can express itself fully to help exchange processes and circulate the information necessary for maintaining homeostasis. Therefore, we must be on constant alert to ensure that the tissues are free of all constraints because these can cause loss of function which, in time, can lead to degenerative phenomena. Thus, by way of example, if the fascial system around a specific joint is exerting sustained pressure over a relatively long time frame, the state of lubrication of the joint will be disturbed. This disturbance will lead to degeneration and, ultimately, to premature wear on the joint.

As described in the previous chapter, the type of fascial testing we advocate involves decoding messages which are sent from the tissues. Once a message has been received and understood, a treatment strategy is chosen based on the most appropriate modality in the light of the information that has been collected.

Modalities and Principles

Here we will define a general principle for the correction of tissue problems. This principle is applicable to all fasciae, with certain provisos for differences among different parts of the body and different pathologies. As we have said, the general principle involves restoring tissue function, that is, first restoring its motility and mobility, which will lead to restoration of normal hemodynamic function and muscle tone.

In Chapter 7 it was explained how contact is first established through our hands, and how this is followed by dialogue. This dialogue makes it possible to decode the messages sent by the fasciae. Treatment is, in effect, an extension of the testing procedure. As we shall see when we turn to specific techniques, most fascial correction is directly induced by the test. Once abnormality has been detected in a tissue, the modus operandi consists of continuing and extending the dialogue with the tissue to provide it with the help it needs to eliminate the restriction. The practitioner who has hitherto remained in receptive mode—a purely passive role—now switches over to a more active one.

For real efficacy, there are two main considerations:

- accuracy
- selecting the most appropriate technique

Accuracy

Accuracy is the key to success in all osteopathic modalities. The more accurate the osteopathic approach, the more effective will be the resolution of tension and the more quickly will the normal physiological functionality of the tissue be restored.

In the vast majority of cases, when a tissue has been damaged, it is incapable of resolving the damage on its own. But, as previously emphasized, fasciae have a capacity for memory and some level of intelligence, and therefore they recognize the problem—it seems as if they are waiting for help from without to give them the means to restore their own natural functionality. The more accurate and suitable the help, the easier it will be for the fascia to 'converse' with the practitioner, and the more likely that the problem will be corrected.

Selecting the most appropriate technique

Determining the most appropriate technique depends on the area to be treated, the type of tissue involved, and the specific pathology or distortion. Efficacy depends on both accuracy and selection of the most appropriate technique. Fascial treatment involves two main corrective modalities:

- induction
- direct treatment

INDUCTION

Principles

Induction follows directly from listening. A positive listening test reveals that a tissue is preferentially attracted towards a particular restriction. All the surrounding forces are focused on this point, which exacerbates the tensions there. Therefore, the technique consists of following the direction of the tensions in all parameters. Sometimes there may be just a single axis of tension, but there may also be others. Tissue re-equilibration must be achieved on the basis of all the various axes, and, if we ignore just one of the several lines of tension present, the therapy will be ineffective because a disrupting factor will persist.

General technical aspects

The general approach to induction is to let the hand find its way to the restriction by listening. Simply finding it in this way eliminates some of the axes of restriction and will therefore also have reduced the forces which apply at that point. Then exert mild pressure over the spot for several seconds, or even up to a couple of minutes, until the relaxation of the tissues is sensed via the hand. Release the pressure and listen again. Cycles of induction and listening are continued until the tissue is free in all of its parameters.

In this technique, when we contact the restriction the second time, we must change the parameters of the axes. This is because, while one axis of tension may have been resolved, another may appear. If we do not continually modify our maneuvers in accordance with the tension vectors that are present, we will end up blocking the motility of the tissues. This will get in the way of the treatment, and correction will then be impossible.

In some patients, you may encounter very extensive adherent restrictions, or very old ones, which are difficult to resolve with simple re-equilibration. In these cases, correction will require a more active kind of help to the tissues. The pressure at the focus of the restriction must be slightly greater in order to induce mild stretching. Once the focal point is engaged, gradually release the pressure slightly, and then stretch again to increase the amplitude of the movement. Repeat these steps five or six times in a row.

The hand can also be used to stretch away from the focal point of a restriction in order to oppose the surrounding tension forces. Then come back to above the focal point to create pressure there, and repeat the same series of steps in other directions a matter of five or six times each way.

As a general rule, when we are pursuing this kind of treatment, the time it will take for the tissues to become free is of the order of three to five minutes. After five minutes, it is usually time to stop, as too much stimulation may induce a response which is counter to that being sought, that is, reinforcement of the pre-existing tensions. When one returns to an area that was recently treated, the amount of improvement is often surprising. What happens in these cases is that the lag time for the response to treatment is increased. Sometimes this lag time can be as long as twenty-four hours, or even a matter of days, depending on the history of the lesion and the capacity of the patient to adapt.

It goes without saying that in the process of induction, as much as in listening, it is vital to respect the rhythm of the patient's tissues. The minute movements that we make should be in harmony with those of the tissues; if they are not, the capacity of the fasciae to respond will be overwhelmed, and only reflex spasms will be induced, to the exclusion of all other responses.

Induction is more suitable for large, true fascial sheets or for generalized equilibrium, while it tends to be less effective for ligaments, the mesenteries, and fascial bands and indurations. When the area to be treated is very extensive, the technique involves placing the hands far apart, thus creating two fixed points around which a whole section of fascia can be manipulated and harmonized. In practice, when a fascia is inhibited, it requires an external stabilization point around which to reinitiate its motility.

DIRECT TREATMENT

Principle

Direct fascial treatment is based on using the tips of one or more fingers to enter into direct contact with the injured area in order to manipulate, stretch, and inhibit it with a view to releasing the restriction. This is mainly applicable to certain specific anatomical features, including the ligaments, mesenteries, modified fascial insertion points, and sections of fasciae in which bands, restrictions, or areas of induration have been detected. Therefore, it is most commonly used for long-standing restrictions and well-established modifications deep in tissues, both of which are situations in which induction is not powerful enough to reestablish normalcy.

Here, as previously discussed, one encounters modifications to viscoelastic properties and changes in fascial structure associated with the appearance of bands (usually with a pearly sheen, and sometimes twisted) or areas of induration (varying from the size of a grain of sand to that of an olive pit). Exchange processes in such tissues are profoundly disturbed, and serious tensions are permanently present, which leads to a vicious cycle of degenerative phenomena.

In these areas, the fascia is overwhelmed and no longer capable of defending itself—it is exhausted. It is not itself capable of overcoming this exhaustion on its own and therefore needs help from without in order to resume the normal physiological functions which were undermined by the original insult.

Therefore, one must use an appropriate technique (e.g., massage or stretching) to 'wake up' the damaged fascial tissue so that it can regain its normal functionality. If left untreated, such 'lethargy' on the part of the tissues can last for years, and, unfortunately, can act as a trigger and focal point for chronic degenerative processes.

In our experience it is always worthwhile to intervene in these situations, even if they have been present for a long time, as some function can always be regained, although perhaps only a very small fraction. For the patients a very small incremental recovery of function can lead to a major improvement in quality of life and sense of well-being.

It is always somewhat surprising to people to realize that sometimes, for unknown reasons, the tissues are able to recover their proper functions and activities even after a long period of dormancy. Everyone has heard of cases of people recovering functions or getting rid of chronic pain after small falls or other minor traumas. We regard these as minor "shocks" to the nervous system that can lead to the reorganization of physiological circuits and pathways. They remind us that one should never give up and that, as long as the patients are willing and interested in getting treatment, we should never regard any case as being hopeless.

Techniques

Direct techniques involve establishing direct contact with the structure to be treated and then exerting pressure or stretching force, the degree of which will vary according to the specific structure or area, the condition of the patient, and the cause of the damage. Gentle contact and very moderate force is required to restore freedom of movement in certain tissues, while others will require firmer contact and relatively strong manipulation in order to 'wake them up,' as will be discussed more later. In certain areas, the pressure exerted can be near the limit of the patient's tolerance—in these cases, it would seem that the pressure required for elimination of the restriction corresponds to the Lewit needle effect. Lewit proposed that the efficacy of an injected drug depends less on the actual agent being administered than on the intensity of pain induced at the injection site, and the accuracy with which the needle (in our case, the finger) is placed at the point of maximum sensitivity.

With respect to pain, it was previously mentioned that it can be a useful indicator, but is often misleading. Damage to the fascia is almost always associated with pain, which is, in some cases, highly acute. It is particularly common in association with fascial bands, isolated spots of induration, and fascial insertion points. When it comes to fascial pathology, pain can be said to be an important diagnostic clue, and that its attenuation or elimination is one of the markers of successful treatment. It should be taken into account, but its intensity should be gauged in light of the nature of the patient, where the damage is located, and the type of injury. It is a fact that some patients tolerate pain relatively well, while the threshold for others is much lower. Pressure that induces significant levels of pain is justified in certain areas (e.g., the plantar aponeurosis), while in others, it should be avoided (e.g., the intertubercular sulcus).

In all cases, if we have settled upon a treatment approach which involves painful pressure, it is unwise to prolong it beyond a certain time or level because excessive pain is likely to induce a response counter to that desired. If the treatment is accurate and performed correctly, all pain from the technique should disappear within a very short period of time. If the treatment is inappropriate or poorly executed, and the fascia reacts violently, residual pain can persist for several days, even if the treated area was originally perfectly silent.

The techniques of direct fascial treatment can be broken down on the basis of five general principles:

- massage pressure
- stretching
- sliding pressure
- the special case of ligaments
- structural techniques

Massage pressure

This is relevant when the zone to be treated consists of a single point or is very small in area, for example, a fascial insertion point or a nodular area.

After the area has been scrupulously examined, apply a greater or lesser degree of pressure, usually with the thumb. At the same time, perform a stretching motion and rotate the thumb as if you were giving a massage (Fig. 8-1). Rather than immediately exerting full pressure, start gently and step it up gradually—wait for the fasciae to open to let you through. For maximum efficacy, despite the pain which you might induce and the pressure you will have to use, it is important to follow the response of the fasciae, which will steadily bring you to maximum pressure.

Maintain the pressure for a few seconds, and then recommence the manipulation, still being guided by the fascia itself. Four or five cycles are often sufficient to induce significant improvement. Similarly, four or five repetitions of a movement are often ideal for the other techniques (apart from structural techniques). Do not repeat more than five times; instead, resume the treatment at a later date if necessary.

The purpose of this form of treatment is to eliminate as much of the induration as possible. A good tip is to imagine that you have between your fingers a friable body which you are steadily reducing to dust. The fascia is exhausted, and the pressure of massage is gradually lifting this exhaustion. The motility and mobility of the fascia are restored, and within a very short time the induration (which appeared to be calcified) disappears.

Fig. 8-1 Direct Technique: Massage Pressure

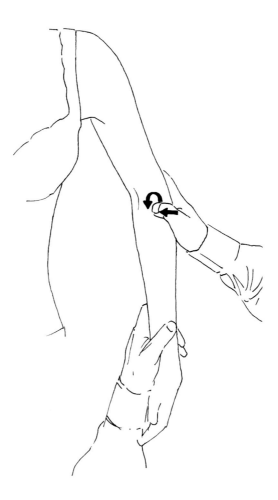

Stretching

These techniques are relevant to fascial bands or areas of fascia of a few centimeters in size. As discussed above, the fascial bands are often extremely tense, with very sharply defined edges.

First, establish the location of both ends of the band and then place the tip of a finger at at each of these two points. Perform traction along the longitudinal axis of the band, taking into account any movement of the underlying fascia (Fig.

8-2). Next, hook one or two fingers around the sharp edge of the band. Steadily increase perpendicular traction, still taking fascial movement into account with longitudinal traction. This second maneuver will be more painful than the first, so it is important to perform the technique with sensitivity so that the pain does not lead to guarding.

Fig. 8-2 Stretching Technique

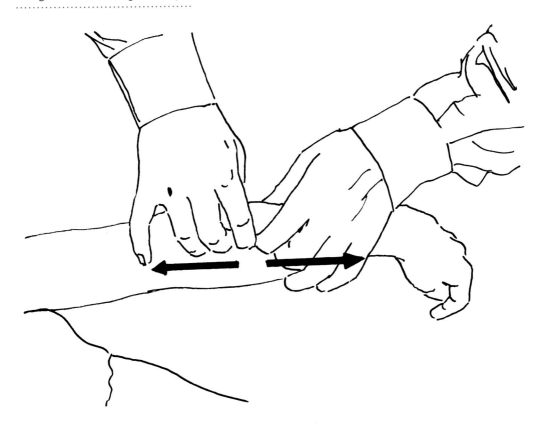

When it comes to working with fasciae (which will usually be in deep regions, or in a cleavage plane between two fasciae), steadily descend into the deeper tissues, either with the fingers of both hands, or with just the thumbs (depending on the size of the area to be treated) until contact. At his point, perform longitudinal traction via opposite movements of the fingers of each hand. Maintaining the longitudinal traction force, next perform traction at right angles to the fascial plane (Fig. 8-3). *Take fascial movements into account during all manipulations.* This applies to all techniques, and won't be mentioned again.

If the tension is superficial and threadlike, simple traction perpendicular to the fibers will usually suffice. In all cases, the goal is to stop the fascial spasm, relieve congestion, and thereby eliminate tension and irritation.

Here, a good tip for successful treatment is to imagine that you have a thick paste which you want to reduce to a thin film so that it can be easily manipulated between the fingers.

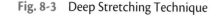
Fig. 8-3 Deep Stretching Technique

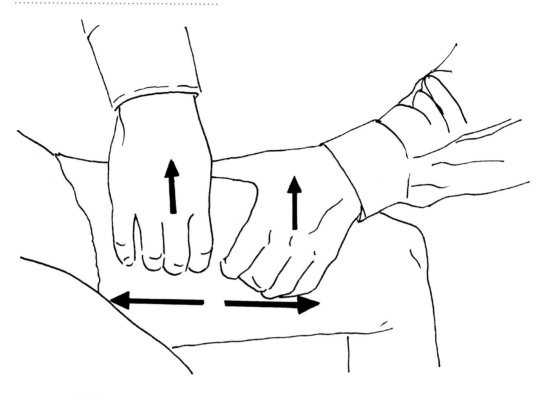

Sliding pressure

These techniques apply to large circular areas which are adherent to the deep periosteum, either over a long length (e.g., the tibial fascia) or following a cleavage fascia.

▶ COVERING AN EXTENSIVE AREA

Slide your finger along the fascia, exerting moderate pressure (Fig. 8-4). A number of different situations are possible:

- If the fascia is abnormally ridged, exert brief pulses of pressure with the thumb to flatten out the ridges and allow passage to the next. This is akin to smoothing out a crumpled piece of paper.
- If you encounter a tense, twisted fascial band, you should still exert brief pulses of pressure, but add a rotational movement in order to restore the fascia to the correct position. This will resolve the tension so that you can proceed with the sliding movement.
- A final possibility is that your thumb may be blocked by a tense, edematous area. In this case, exert slightly more pressure and, if necessary, some rotation until the fascia relaxes to allow continuation of the sliding displacement.

▶ ALONG A CLEAVAGE FASCIA

As in the preceding case, the technique consists of sliding the thumb along

Fig. 8-4   Treating an Extensive Fascial Restriction

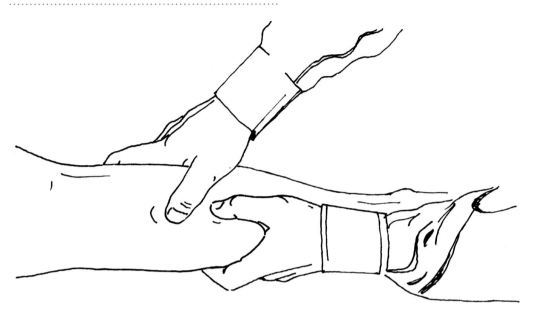

the cleavage plane between two different fasciae. You will meet certain places which are more tense and painful. Stop there and exert greater pressure, coupled with rotation or perpendicular traction.

▶ OVER A CIRCULAR AREA

Circular restrictions are often encountered where the fascia is in direct contact with the periosteum. The area is edematous and raised, with its center over the connection of the restriction to the periosteum.

Apply sliding pressure all around the edge of the area, and then gradually progress towards the center (*Fig. 8-5a*). Next, make contact at the restriction and, while exerting fairly strong pressure, make stretching displacements in all directions. Finally, with the feeling of being adhered to the tissues, you will induce a rotation and then stretch primarily in the direction of the main restrictions, which is usually laterally (*Fig. 8-5b*).

The goal of all these techniques is the same as in the other cases. A useful tip here is to imagine that you are holding between your fingers an ice cube which is gradually melting—always seek fluidity.

Ligaments

By virtue of their special functions, ligaments are a class apart and require specific treatment modalities. As a general rule, make contact with the thumb and then exert pressure at right angles to the direction of the fibers of the ligament. If possible, try to make an additional contact using the palm of the other hand in the most suitable location to enable the two hands to work together. One hand will exert a stretching pressure and the other will exert a similar stretching pressure, but will change position slightly in order to work in all the necessary planes.

Fig. 8-5a Treating a Circular Restriction

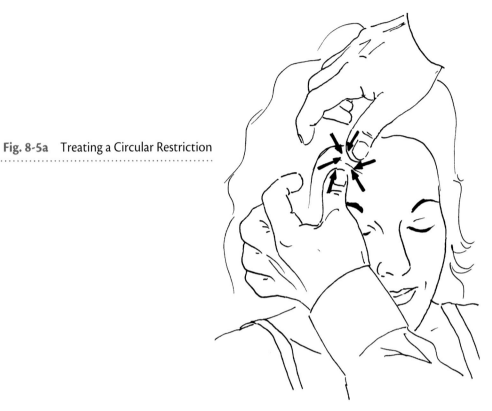

Fig. 8-5b Treating a Circular Restriction

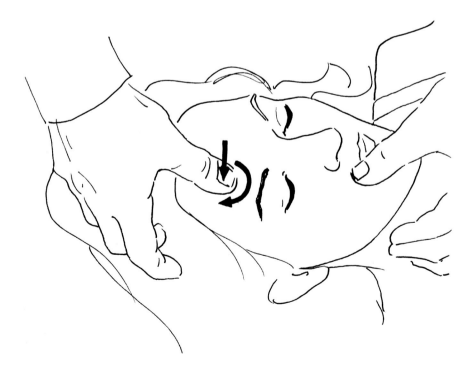

If possible, after establishing contact with the ligament, it is a good idea to try to move the body around the ligament in order to allow it to relax. For example, when treating the sacrotuberous ligament, you should contact the middle of the ligament with one thumb, and then stretch the ligament perpendicular to its axis. At the same time, the other hand is placed on the sacrum near the insertion, and increases the traction by following the direction of the fibers of the fascia.

When damaged, certain ligaments become very tense and feel heavily indurated on palpation. It is necessary to restore the elasticity of such ligaments. This kind of strategy is reflected in the iliolumbar ligament technique below.

Structural techniques

I use the term 'structural techniques' to refer to those that are more forceful and have a greater amplitude of motion than techniques based on listening and induction. Structural techniques remain the ideal modality for treating fascial problems, especially those of the short, deep fascial elements which are difficult to access by palpation. In most cases, structural lesions are first and foremost fascial lesions. In a large proportion, somatic dysfunction can only be sustained by the surrounding soft tissues, which gradually change, become fibrotic, and adhere to an ever greater extent to the area of dysfunction. This is inevitably accompanied by ongoing degenerative processes.

Obviously, if the lesion involves the vertebral fasciae, it will be very difficult to gain access to the deep fasciae and their extensions, such as the many joint ligaments. Moreover, if the lesion is long standing, it will be under such high tension that calcification may ensue. Structural techniques are the most suitable, and definitely the most effective, in these situations. These techniques involve inducing rapid stretching of the tissues to prevent their spasm. This induces relaxation, which will in turn restore free movement to the joint.

Not all structural lesions are exclusively maintained by a fascial process. The tibiotarsal, metacarpophalangeal, and interphalangeal articulations in particular seem to be subject to some other kind of process. Of course, the lesion is associated with a tissular component, but resolution of the tissue problem does not necessarily correct the lesion as a whole. In practice, in these particular joints there is superimposed a phenomenon of articular 'vacuum' which sticks the various elements of the joint together, rather like a suction cup. As long as we have not succeeded in freeing up the joint and regenerating some pressure within it, it can never be fully functional.

Specific Techniques

We are not going to systematically cover all the techniques applicable to the various fasciae. Rather, we will focus on the general principles of treating fasciae, as introduced in the preceding section, by looking at certain particularly pertinent examples drawn from different parts of the body.

LOWER LIMB

Plantar aponeurosis

As a result of the many distortions to which the foot is subject, seriously abnormal tension is common in the plantar aponeurosis. Such tension will inhibit foot function, can prevent successful therapy based on structural techniques, and is sometimes the cause of a pathological heel spur.

With the patient prone and their leg bent, penetrate deeply to feel the cord-like structure which supports the plantar arch. First, apply sliding pressure, concentrating on the area which is most sensitive. Then hook the ligament with the tips of the fingers and stretch it in a transverse direction (Fig. 8-6).

This technique is extremely painful, so one must first warn the patient and obtain their permission. Never exceed the limit of tolerable pain. Given these basic precautions, the manipulation should be firm but brief. Results are often very fast—in the vast majority of cases, one or two sessions will suffice, although more may be necessary if the lesion is of long standing and the original injury was very serious.

Fig. 8-6   Treatment of the Plantar Aponeurosis

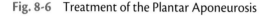
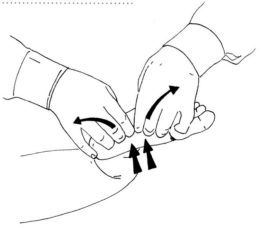

If there is a pathological heel spur originating from the calcaneal tuberosity, treat the plantar aponeurosis first, and then concentrate your efforts on the tuberosity itself, applying pressure with rotation. Then treat the fascia around the heel, and ascend back upward along the achilles tendon as far as the calf, where tension most commonly resides in the cleavage plane between the two bellies of the gastrocnemius muscles. Again, the pain from treatment should not last too long. Often the process becomes reduced and sometimes disappears altogether.

Tibial fascia

The fascia which directly invests the tibia is often involved in lower limb lesions and is often key to successful treatment of knee and ankle problems.

This is treated with the patient supine and their knee either extended or bent, with the foot resting on the table. Apply sliding pressure along the fascia with stretching, massaging, and rotation at any points of restriction. Ascend back up to the medial tibial plateau (Fig. 8-7). Once all restrictions have been relaxed, it will be possible to slide the finger all the way along the fascia without encountering any impediments to progress or inducing any pain.

Treating the tibial fascia is often key to a problem of a sore ankle associated with difficulty with respect to plantar flexion. Following distortion, the sudden stretching entailed by an inappropriate movement is entirely absorbed by the tibial fascia. Although this preserves the ligaments of the ankle, it can create tension and induce restrictions of the tibial fascia itself.

Fig. 8-7 Treatment of the Tibial Fascia

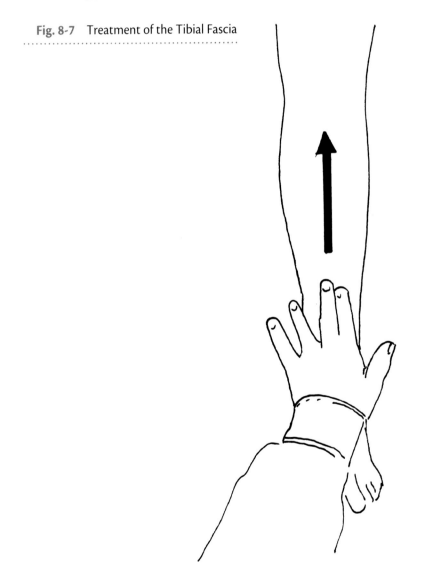

It should also be pointed out that the tibial fascia is a common area to which gynecological problems are projected. This causes changes in fascial reflexes, usually around the middle of the lateral aspect of the tibia, and around the medial condyle, in the form of edema, infiltration, and pain. Treating such areas often has an impact on the underlying gynecological problem.

Sometimes the function of the entire tibial fascia is impaired without there being any specific focal points of restriction. The treatment will consist of listening and induction: either in a general (also known as global) mode, by placing one hand over the lower part of the tibia and the other over the upper part; or by adopting a more localized approach, gradually moving closer and closer to the localized structures. Once this has released, you should finish by using a general technique that affects the entire fascia.

Thigh

In the vast majority of cases, problems here involve just the lateral or just the medial thigh.

Lateral thigh

These are distortions involving the fascia lata. With the patient supine and their legs stretched out, use the tips of two or three fingers to apply sliding pressure along the iliotibial tract (Fig. 8-8). You will often encounter a rippling in the tissues, sort of like a corrugated roof. You must steadily work to reduce the intensity of the rippling, one ridge at a time.

Fig. 8-8 Treatment of the Lateral Fascia of the Thigh

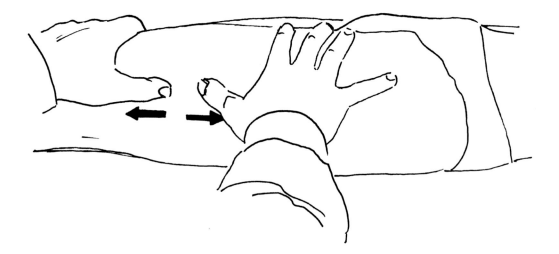

Painful points will be encountered all along the fascia in the form of nodules—these can be reduced by massage and rotational movements. Here, as in all cases of fascial treatment, effective therapy will result in reduced tension, major reduction in the associated pain, and of course improved functionality.

Medial thigh

With the patient supine, knee and hip slightly bent, the practitioner takes up a position to the side of the patient, with their knee on the table. Rest the lateral aspect of the patient's thigh against your own thigh. Place the finger tips of both hands along the cleavage plane between the adductor muscles, and then apply a stretching pressure (Fig. 8-9). If there is a more serious restriction, place both thumbs on the upper edge of the adductor muscles and perform a transverse stretching movement, pushing towards the table.

Fig. 8-9   Treatment of the Medial Fascia of the Thigh

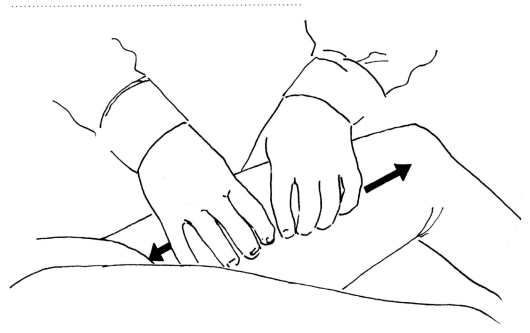

Sciatic nerve fascia

We will finish with the lower limb by talking about treatment of the sciatic nerve fascia. In the previous chapter, it was mentioned that this can be the site of chronic irritation, and the reason for the persistence of sciatica. Sometimes problems with this fascia can even be the cause of sciatica.

Pertinent to this is an anecdote which is significant in our approach to fasciae. Just about all osteopaths in Europe have had patients who have reported visiting some kind of bone-setter who "put their nerves back where they belong" and, in the case of sciatica especially, sometimes with spectacular results. The technique actually consists of using the thumb—with the patient either prone or standing—to trace the path of the sciatic nerve all the way back to the buttocks, or even to trace the tension up through the lumbodorsal fascia as far as the cervical vertebrae. Of course, in nearly all cases, the patient retains an indelible memory of the thumb lightly caressing the area to be treated and leaving a sensation which took a long time to disappear. Is the patient's sciatica improved every time?

This has always surprised us and we sought an explanation for many years. In the end, the explanation is a simple one, yet it is a profound understanding of anatomy which provides it. The sciatic nerve is invested by a fascia, and tension in the nerve inevitably causes irritation of the fascia. The bone-setter is not working the nerve, but rather the fascia. This is an example of how traditional remedies nearly always have some kind of foundation in truth.

The 'stress' induced by the technique seems to 'wake' the amnesic fascia up, which suddenly realizes that its function is impaired. The strong stimulus banished the exhaustion and restored the memory of the normal physiological situation. We have adapted this principle and have often used it with success.

The patient is prone. After you have identified the restricted area (which is usually around the middle of the thigh, as described earlier), introduce the finger tips of both hands deeply and then perform transverse, longitudinal stretching (Fig. 8-10). Move down the length of the fascia as far as the calf, at which point it will be more comfortable for you if you place one thigh on the table and apply pressure above the patient's bent leg. Regardless of your position, you then proceed to stretch or use pressure to inhibit the specific point (Fig. 8-11).

It is not necessary, in the vast majority of cases, to use such strong pressure that the patient feels pain. Nor, of course, is it necessary to work the entire lower limb with the thumb, because the same result can be obtained by the much gentler procedure.

Fig. 8-10   Treatment of the Sciatic Nerve Fascia

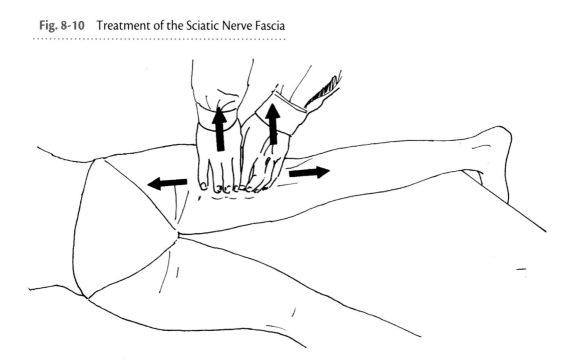

Fig. 8-11   Treatment of the Sciatic Nerve Fascia

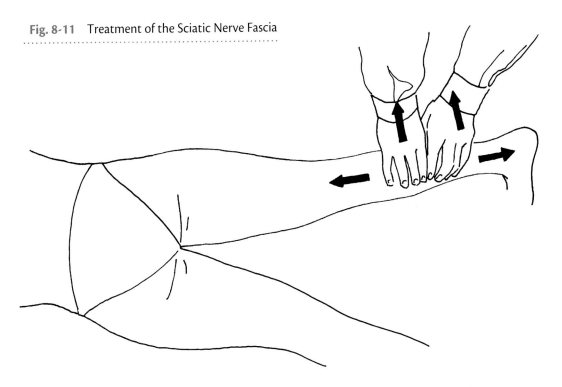

After such an approach, we often observe improved function, notably attenuation or disappearance of Lasègue's sign. Of course, this technique is not the only treatment modality for sciatica, and is always coupled with a scrupulous examination for possible causes. Moreover, it often needs to be combined with other techniques.

PELVIS

We will not go into how to release the sacrotuberous and sacrospinous ligaments or the piriformis muscle in any detail because these techniques are familiar to all. However, we would emphasize that the sacrospinous ligament is often a key factor in problems of the pelvis and the lower limb. It should therefore be inspected as a routine procedure. We will concentrate instead on two specific techniques for:

- the fasciae of the gluteus muscles
- the iliolumbar and lumbosacral ligaments

Fasciae of the gluteus muscles

These fasciae cover an extensive area and are quite active, especially in the standing position.

With the patient prone use the thumb to apply sliding pressure. Alternatively, a stretching or inhibition technique can be used. Treatment should be applied to the following areas:

- the line of insertion along the iliac crest where fascial bands and nodular areas are often encountered (Fig. 8-12)
- the fasciae investing the various muscles which traverse obliquely and inferolaterally; to be effective, you must penetrate deeply between the various bundles of fibers
- the insertion line of the fascia all the way along the lateral edge of the sacrum as far as the contact with the bone. Fascial bands and nodular areas are often encountered here as well

Fig. 8-12   Treatment of the Gluteal Fasciae

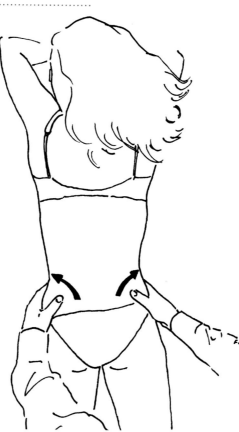

Better results are often obtained if the technique is performed with the patient standing. For example, to treat the fascia on the right, stand behind and support the patient. Pass your left arm below that of the patient, and encircle them. Then, while supporting the patient on your left arm, translate the pelvis towards the left as you incline the chest towards the right. This will relieve the tension at the level of the fascia and help your work with your right hand.

Iliolumbar ligament

This tight, rope-like structure is found between the transverse muscles of L4 and

L5 and the iliac crest. It is essential that this be treated if you want to normalize the lumbosacral junction.

As previously discussed, this technique depends on the patient standing erect; it is not effective with the patient prone because this ligament must support weight in order to be ready for treatment. Taking, by way of example, treatment of the ligament on the right-hand side:

The patient stands with their legs slightly apart. The practitioner should take up a position behind the patient and in contact with their back. Pass your left arm under that of the patient to encircle and stabilize them. Position your right thumb over the middle of the ligament and exert pressure at right angles.

Very often, even mild pressure proves excessively painful and it is virtually impossible to depress the ligament, which feels as if it is calcified. Therefore, for this ligament, it is often necessary to mobilize the whole body to reintegrate the ligament into the general layout. To do this, flex the patient (to a greater or lesser extent) by simply pulling back a small distance on their pelvis. The patient's feet should not move at any time during this manipulation. Then bring the patient into right sidebending and then left rotation (Fig. 8-13). Throughout all of these manipulations, maintain pressure on the ligament with the right thumb, the amount of pressure depending on the degree of associated pain.

You must repeatedly readjust the position of the body around the ligament as the technique progresses. Come back to the original position before reintroducing the various parameters.

The difficulty with this technique is related to the fact that the patient is afraid of falling and tends to tense up, which makes the procedure impossible. Therefore, it is important to carefully explain what is going to happen and what is expected of the patient. Then proceed only as long as he or she is totally relaxed. In order to reassure the patient, make sure they are being firmly supported, and for extra reassurance, you can bring your left leg round in contact with the side of the patient's, which provides a second support plane. This can be used as a first line treatment, but for maximum efficacy, it should be undertaken after other techniques, for example, after articular techniques on the soft tissues of the pelvis, or after structural correction.

When executed correctly, this technique results in a major improvement in the capacity for anterior flexion, which will facilitate the process of normalization.

Lumbosacral ligament

This technique is more or less the same as the one described above for the iliolumbar ligament. Place one thumb over the upper part of the sulcus and put the patient into a position of extension, right sidebending, and left rotation. It should be mentioned that this ligament is not involved nearly as often as the iliolumbar ligament.

Fig. 8-13   Treatment of the Iliolumbar Ligament

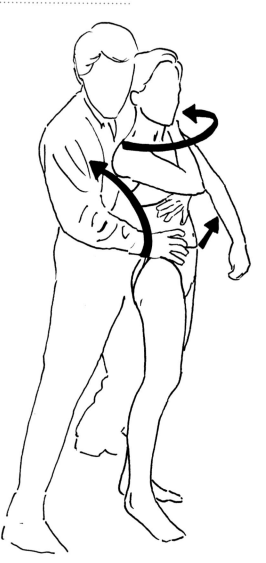

THORACIC REGION

Thoracolumbar fascia

One of the quintessential fascial regions, this one is prone to many fascial problems.

It is treated with the patient prone. Starting at the sacrum, apply a sliding pressure, moving up as far as the cervical vertebrae (Fig. 8-14). You will encounter fascial bands, nodules, and circular bundles of fibers which are both extremely tense and very extensive.

Fig. 8-14   Treatment of the Thoracolumbar Fascia

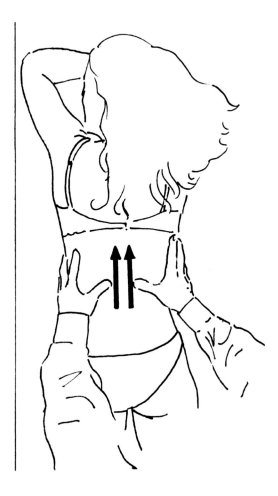

Once you have reached the interscapular region, you will often encounter tensions running in an oblique direction towards the scapulas. The posterior face of the scapula is often a focus for fascial tension, both above and below the process.

To treat these, apply a sliding pressure in an oblique direction towards the shoulder (Fig. 8-15). Isolate the tensions between the muscular bundles and isolate the nodular zones, some of which will be like very tense, hypersensitive balls of tissue. Treat these with stretching, pressure, rotation, and inhibition. Do not forget to apply sliding pressure all along the lateral edge of the scapula, where distortion is common (Fig. 8-16).

Treatment of the thoracic region is sometimes more effective with the patient seated. In this position the force of gravity can be of help. In elderly patients who are difficult to move and for whom prudence is the watchword, using this technique with the patient seated is usually sufficient for lumbosacral problems. It can be employed by itself with immediate, long-lasting results.

Fig. 8-15 Treatment of the Scapular Fasciae

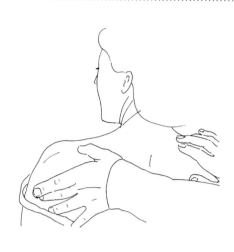

Fig. 8-16 Treatment of the Lateral Scapular Fasciae

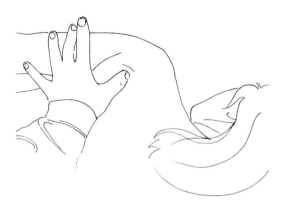

Posterior fasciae

Certain individuals suffer from generalized tension of the posterior fasciae, with difficulty bending forwards. If they are lying down and one of their lower limbs is raised, the flexion angle will be very restricted and pain will soon be induced. A general fascial technique can quickly improve the patient's condition—this technique is equivalent to a lumbar roll, but with no local specificity.

With the patient lying on their side, the practitioner stands facing the patient. Bring the upper part into mild posterior rotation by anterior and cephalad traction on the extremity that is in contact with the table. The leg on the table is maintained in a straight position, while the other one is flexed and dangled off the table.

Contact is made with one elbow on the upper part of the thorax and the other on the pelvis. Introduce some tension by increasing the rotation and adding longitudinal traction (Fig. 8-17). At the same time, using your foot, hook the leg off the table so as to bring it into flexion and adduction, thereby increasing the tension. Make sure that it remains as straight as possible throughout this procedure (Fig. 8-18). A variant involves the practitioner positioning him or herself behind the patient's leg from the outset.

The final part of the technique involves performing a rapid stretch by means of a non-specific thrust. Both arms execute a longitudinal stretch, while the left leg is used to accentuate the flexion adduction of the patient's lower limb. This technique should be performed on both sides and the resulting improvement in mobility should be significant, immediate, and long-lasting.

Fig. 8-17   General Treatment of Posterior Fasciae: Movement of Trunk

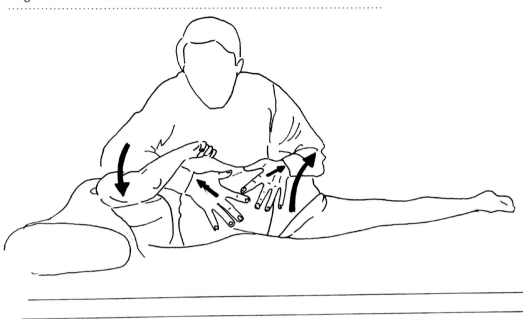

Fig. 8-18   General Treatment of Posterior Fasciae: Movement of Leg

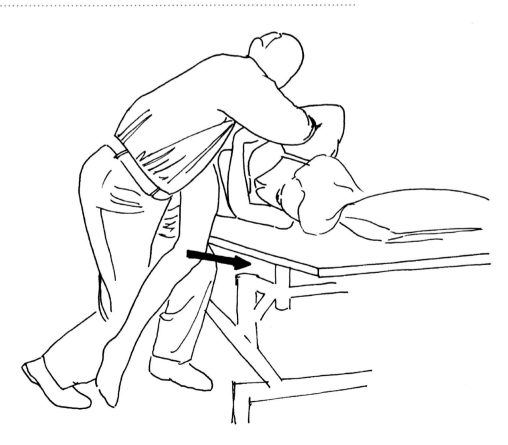

VENTRAL REGION

The ventral region is divided into two different parts, namely, the thorax and the abdomen, which are separated by the diaphragm. The treatment of abdominal fasciae involves the anterior vertebral ligament and the viscera—classic fascial areas. The superficial abdominal fasciae are rarely involved in pathology. We will follow this with descriptions of treatments for the diaphragm and thorax. For the latter, most treatments are directed at the sternum.

Anterior longitudinal ligament

The patient is supine, legs bent, and feet resting on the table. The practitioner takes up a position to the side of the patient and, using the fingers of both hands, gradually depresses the linea alba to make contact with the ligament. After exerting mild pressure, execute a longitudinal stretching movement by moving the hands away from one another (Fig. 8-19). Follow this with a transverse stretch.

This technique must be performed gently and should be avoided if its execution presents any problem. It is often useful and effective in patients with chronic low back pain or sciatica. Remember not to go above the aortic bifurcation.

Fig. 8-19 Treatment of the Anterior Longitudinal Ligament

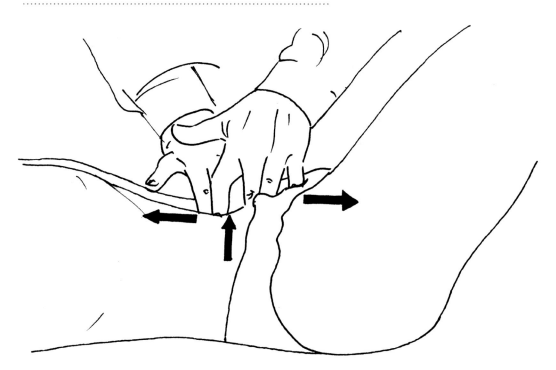

Viscera

It is not at all our intention to review all the visceral techniques, as this has been done comprehensively in many other texts, primarily those of Jean-Pierre Barral. We would only point out that fascial techniques are just as applicable to the viscera. In fact, visceral treatment is nothing more or less than a kind of fascial treatment.

In this region, listening and induction is systematically combined with direct treatment. As a general rule, it is best to begin with listening and induction and proceed to direct treatment if necessary. This can then be followed by another round of listening and induction as a way of finishing.

If there is any part of the body in which passage through the various levels of fascia must be done with caution and gentleness, it is the abdomen. Always wait until the fasciae let you through and never, under any circumstances, try to break through a resistant barrier. As a general rule, the listening and induction phase will involve sliding the hand towards the restriction, maintaining some degree of pressure there, and then, if necessary, slightly increasing the level of pressure to induce some stretching. Then return to the starting position and repeat the operation.

Although you will often find an axis of tension or a preferred direction of movement, always bear in mind that re-equilibration must include all three spatial planes, and that if one plane is favored, it must be constantly readjusted with respect to the others if the technique is to be successful. Progress can only be made by moving with the fasciae. It should be enough to follow them and then make them work with a very slight change.

If the techniques of listening and induction prove insufficient, you must proceed to direct treatment. The principle is the same as for any other fascia, but more caution should be exercised. It will be necessary to penetrate deep into the abdomen, and this can only be done with the consent of the fasciae. You must wait as long as necessary for the chance to pass, and it is vital to follow the movement of the fasciae at all times. All this means that you must overcome any desire to get ahead of what the fasciae will allow.

The actual techniques are based on stretching, pressure, rotation, and inhibition. The fascial bands mainly correspond to the mesentery, the fascias of Toldt and Treitz, and even the vessels in the case of real adhesions. Nodules are particularly common around the sphincters (the pyloric sphincter, sphincter of Oddi, and the iliocecal valve).

Diaphragm

Both fascial continuation and fascia itself, the importance of the diaphragm in human physiology has already been discussed. Therefore, it should be understood how important it is that its movement should be free and unencumbered.

General technique

The patient is supine with their legs bent and feet resting on the table. The practitioner takes up a position to the side of the patient, facing cephalad. With hands spread open wide, make as much contact as possible with the lower ribs, with the thumbs pointing towards the xiphoid process (Fig. 8-20).

Focusing on both mobility and motility, first equilibrate one hemithorax at a time, and then reharmonize them with respect to each other. By the time this is done, the diaphragm and its related structures should be able to move feely in all spatial planes.

Fig. 8-20   Treatment of the Diaphragm: Global Technique

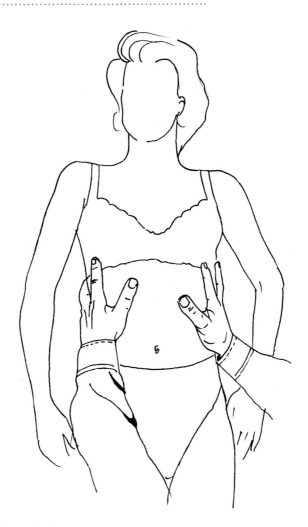

Muscular technique

With the patient and the practitioner in the same positions as above, place both hands on one side of the thorax with the thumbs penetrating between the ribs to contact the muscle insertions. Gradually advance the thumbs as cephalad as possible. Correct any restriction encountered with stretching and inhibition pressure by moving the thumbs in opposite directions (Fig. 8-21). Then proceed to treat the other side of the thorax.

Fig. 8-21   Treatment of the Diaphragm: Muscular Technique

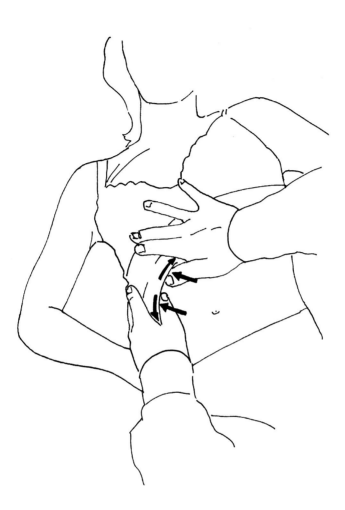

This technique should be followed up by a generalized reharmonization procedure. Since the pillars of the diaphragm are not directly accessible, they are more amenable to the structural technique that mobilizes the lumbar vertebrae to which they attach. Never elicit pain when applying this second technique, because it will immediately trigger a reflex spasm which will push the fingers out.

Sternum

Again, in this region, the fascia is in direct contact with the bone. Moreover, in the deeper area is the pericardium. As previously mentioned, this is particularly sensitive to stress and so is commonly subject to fascial distortion. Fascial bands and nodular areas are very common in this region, particularly in the central portion, and secondarily on the sides and at the apex of the sternum. Work on the sternum can significantly improve palpitations, tachycardia, stress, and anxiety.

Induction

With the patient supine the practitioner takes up a position to the side or at the head of the patient. Place one hand over the sternum, making as much contact as possible, and exerting a sucker effect. Here, the common problems are twisting, posterior attraction, axial tightening of the sternum, or some combination of these. The general therapeutic principle is the same as anywhere else: starting at a favored axis, re-harmonize the sternum in all its parameters so that it once again 'floats' completely freely (Fig. 8-22).

Fig. 8-22 Induction of the Sternum

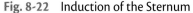

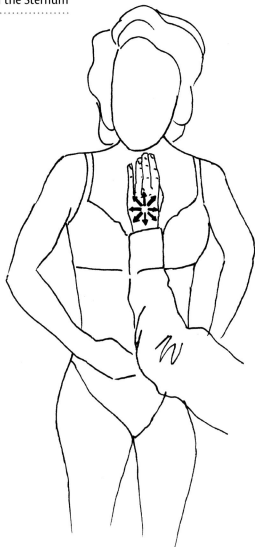

Direct technique

With the patient still in the same position, apply sliding pressure all along the length of the sternum, both its median segment and its lateral edges, in the manner of all direct techniques. Here it is particularly useful to follow up this technique with listening and induction.

Often, acute pain will result and it is important to correctly modulate the pressure. If inappropriate pressure is applied, the patient may continue to feel pain (usually a burning or insect bite type of pain) for several days. If the pressure used was really excessive, the pain may persist for a matter of weeks, which risks becoming a genuine inconvenience for the patient and a possible source of anxiety.

UPPER LIMB

The upper limb is working almost all the time and we consider it as something of a special case. This is based on its morphology, how its fasciae function, and its responses. Despite its non-stop activity, it presents fewer problems than other parts of the body, apart from its root, which, by contrast, seems to accumulate problems, the reasons for which we have already discussed. It responds poorly to techniques based on listening and induction, but is relatively amenable to direct techniques.

We will deal separately with techniques for:

- the forearm
- the elbow
- the arm
- the shoulder

Forearm

Fascial bands are less common here. More common are tensions in the cleavage planes in the shape of straight or twisted ropes. Nodules are also common and are often very painful.

With the patient supine, apply sliding pressure to the anterior or posterior face of the forearm, moving up as far as the elbow. As a rule, this sliding will bring you towards the medial or lateral epicondyle along two favored axes which are the most common sites for restrictions, especially on the lateral (radial) side. In general, the hardest working region is along the edges of the brachioradialis muscle, especially its anteromedial edge.

When manipulating the medial (ulnar) part, the pressure should be stronger. If the tension there is strong, it will be terminated in the lower part by the pronator quadratus and in the upper part by the obliquely oriented muscles. This will sometimes feel like a hypertrophic ball and will be very painful.

As you advance, feel the tense fibers running longitudinally and try to stretch them in a perpendicular direction (Fig. 8-23). Similarly, feel the circular areas deeper down and correct them using massage, rotation, and inhibition.

Working on the forearm often elicits pain. Sometimes, pain-inducing degrees of force must be used in order to guarantee efficacy, therefore always forewarn the patient and obtain their consent. Given this, the results can be truly impressive.

Fig. 8-23   Treatment of the Fasciae of the Forearm

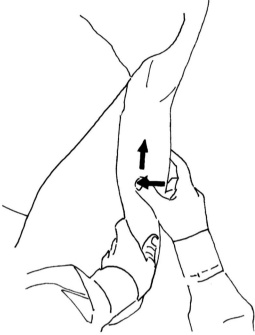

These techniques for the forearm are particularly effective for cramps in the hands, morning stiffness of the fingers, pain when using the fingers, and radicular arthritis. When they are combined with work on the thumb, they can be effective in patients with carpal canal problems and, of course, with any kind of tendinitic irritation in the forearm or the elbow. Shoulder problems sometime respond to fascial treatment of the forearm. This just requires that one follow the chain of fascial elements.

Elbow

The elbow represents a relay point between the anterolateral and posterolateral fascial chains of the forearm, and the lateral chain of the upper arm. In this region, the fasciae are particularly hard-working and the most common problem is tendinitis on the lateral side. Tendinitis of the medial epichondyle is much less common. Osteopaths are often consulted for epicondylitis, which responds well to fascial treatment.

The treatment is done with the patient supine. Before you arrive at the actual elbow, you must treat the fascial chain of the forearm. In the vast majority of cases, this chain is continuous with the medial anterior edge of the brachioradialis muscle.

Next comes the epicondyle, where fascial bands of nodular insertion areas are common. These can act as foci of calcification. Exert firm inhibition pressure on the problem point and, if necessary, stretch the fibers (8-24). The success of the technique seems to be proportional to the amount of pressure used. As a result, the technique is often associated with particularly acute pain and should therefore be accomplished quickly. For best results, you must extend work on the elbow with treatment of the lateral chain of the arm.

Fig. 8-24   Treatment of the Fasciae of the Elbow

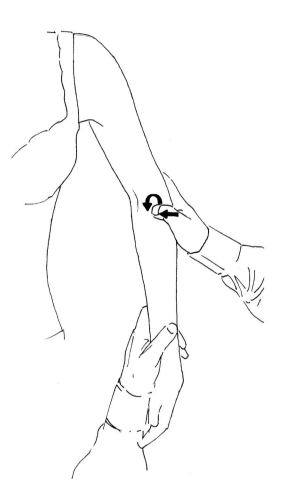

In general, functional improvement is immediate. As in every case, the difficult issue is how to gauge the degree of needed pressure. Above and beyond a certain level, more pressure is useless and can even exacerbate the symptoms. In practice, the amount of pressure needed depends on the etiology of the tendonitis, and pain-inducing pressure is quite inappropriate in some forms. Your judgment must depend on careful questioning of the patient and your own experience.

Arm

In the arm, most problems involve the lateral chain, as this is where most of the tensions focus.

With the patient supine, exert a sliding pressure from the elbow up to the deltoid 'V' (Fig. 8-25). Here, there will be longitudinal fascial bands with, in some cases, a circular area of infiltration which can be treated by massage and rotation.

The deltoid V is often a focus of hypertrophy, which should be treated with inhibition pressure and transverse stretching. Then continue either forwards or backwards, or even via the middle of the deltoid, depending on the direction of the tension.

Fig. 8-25 Treatment of the Fasciae of the Arm

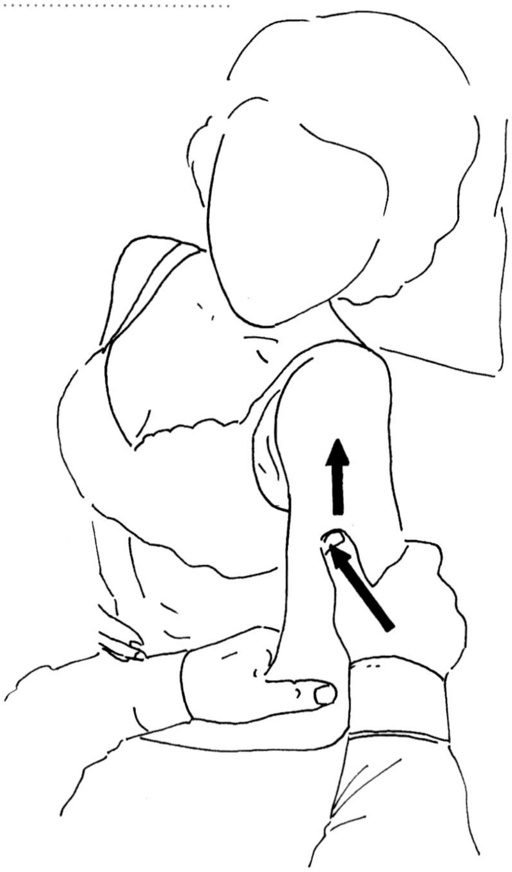

Shoulder

The shoulder is the ultimate fascial junction where a large number of different aponeuroses and other fascial elements meet. The fasciae around the scapula have to work very hard, and the treatment of this region is extremely critical, requiring extensive exploration. In addition, in strictly local terms, fascial treatment can be of enormous benefit.

The patient should be seated, as the effect of the weight of the arm is necessary for a good result, because it provides some traction. The practitioner takes up a position behind the patient, supporting their back. Apply a sliding pressure along the cleavage planes of the deltoid muscle, moving towards the deltoid 'V'

(Fig. 8-26). You will often encounter deep fascial bands, which should be treated by inhibition pressure and transverse stretching.

Fig. 8-26   Treatment of the Fasciae of the Shoulder

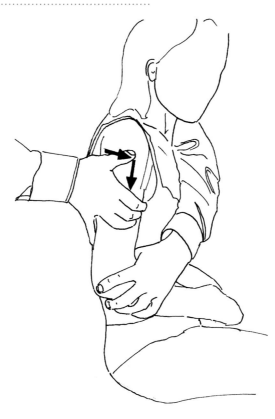

Next, treat the area around the scapula using the same techniques as above. Sometimes it is worth checking the upper end-point of the medial brachial chain by introducing the thumb into the axillary fossa. Do not ignore the fascial chain of the upper limb, but for this, as previously discussed, the patient should be supine.

As with everywhere else, treatment of the fasciae of the shoulder elicits pain, but, in this region, it is especially important to know how to control the amount of pain you are causing. Too much pressure will induce too strong a reaction, which will end up by exacerbating the symptoms. The intertubercular sulcus, often a focus for extremely painful irritation, warrants special caution and must never be subject to exaggerated pressure.

NECK

Shoulder girdle

With the patient supine the practitioner takes up a position behind the patient's head. Place your thumbs in front of the anterior edge of the trapezius muscle, pointing towards the first rib, and close to the vertebral axis. Rest your index fingers on, and parallel to, the subclavicular fasciae. Press with the palms of the hands on the lateral clavicles and the apexes of the shoulders. The middle fingers rests on the pectoral muscle while the ring and little fingers are on the shoulders and deltoid muscles (Fig. 8-27).

Exert mild pressure with the thumbs. Often, one side will be more resistant than the other and may feel like a round ball which is difficult to depress. Perform listening and induction, with the thumbs following the movement of the tissues.

Fig. 8-27   Treatment of the Fasciae of the Shoulder Girdle

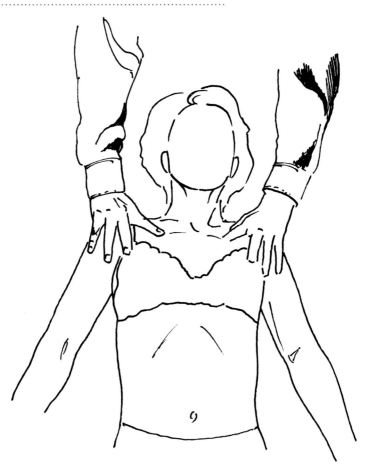

Next, you can increase the pressure and combine it with light rotation and stretching in the appropriate directions. The 'ball' will gradually resolve under the action of the thumb, and the patient's pain in response to the pressure will disappear.

At the same time, the fingers should be controlling the tensions at the level of the shoulders. If this tension is too great, perform listening and induction in order to bring it back to normal. This technique should not involve any heavy pressure and should be completely painless. Relaxation should occur within no more than three minutes, at most.

You will often find major tension around the shoulder which actually prevents this technique. Should this be the case, perform a *direct long lever technique*. This is done by supporting the patient's head very securely with one hand under the base of the skull, and additional support from your abdomen. Your other hand is placed on the apex of the shoulder. Exert pressure using the hand at the shoulder while simultaneously sidebending and rotating the cervical vertebrae toward the opposite side. The success of this technique depends on sidebending along with the correct level of flexion or extension and the right degree of rotation in order to obtain the maximum about of tension.

This technique also represents a generalized treatment for the lateral fasciae of the neck. When this is finished, perform the preceding technique.

Cartilages

The cartilages of the neck have significant fascial connections and often require treatment.

With the patient supine the practitioner is positioned on either side of the patient's head. We will use the right side in the examples below. This technique requires sequential operations, starting with the general and proceeding to the more specific.

First, place your left hand on the patient's forehead, with the fingers of your right hand placed along the left edge of the throat. Rotate the head to the left while translating the throat straight to the right (Fig. 8-28). As the technique proceeds, slightly increase the pressure from the right hand, especially at the point of maximum tension. Then rotate the head to the right and, using the thumb, push the cartilages out towards the left.

Next, treat the hyoid bone following the general principle of inducing mild stretching away from the focus of resistance, gradually increasing the force as you continue (Fig. 8-29).

Stage three involves taking the hyoid bone between the thumb and index finger of your left hand and the thyroid cartilage between the thumb and index finger of your right hand. Perform counter-translation of the two cartilages in order to put the point of resistance under tension (Fig. 8-30). Proceed in the same way to stage four and treat the thyroid and cricoid cartilages in a similar manner.

This technique can soon become extremely painful and is frankly distressing for certain patients. Therefore, it is important to increase the pressure very gradually. When performed correctly, it can be of great benefit to patients with a sore throat, hoarseness, or irritation, or whose voice has changed in some way.

We once treated a patient who, following an inappropriate movement, suddenly found that they could no longer sing in tune. Cartilage treatment to the neck immediately restored the patient's voice to normal. We have also treated an opera singer who, whenever she had a stiff neck, could no longer reach the high notes. Again, a simple cartilage treatment resolved the problem. We have seen many, many cases like this.

Cervicopleural ligaments

The patient is supine, with the practitioner stationed behind their head. Take the base of the skull in your hand and support the patient's head on your abdomen. With the thumb of the other hand, make contact with the ligament to be treated. Sidebend the head ipsilaterally while monitoring the relaxation of the ligament with the thumb and exerting mild pressure there to take up any slack.

Readjust the position in all planes with the thumb maintaining the tension of the ligament. Usually you will need to slightly flex, extend, rotate, and sidebend to get the maximum effect. Wait until relaxation is complete, with constant readjustment of position.

The final phase involves maintaining contact with the ligament and bringing the cervical column into sidebending towards the opposite side (Fig. 8-31). This technique warrants a high degree of caution because of the structures associated with the pleural dome. If the manipulation is poorly executed, it is not uncommon to induce redness of the face, dizziness, and even mild malaise.

Fig. 8-28   General Treatment of the Axis of the Neck

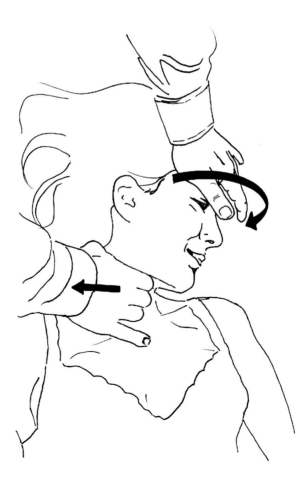

Fig. 8-29   Hyoid Treatment

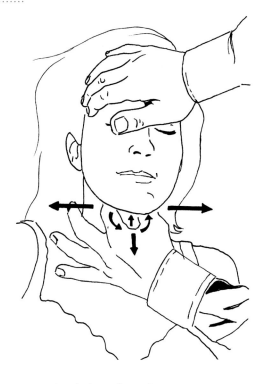

Fig. 8-30   Treatment of the Hyoid and Thyroid Cartilage

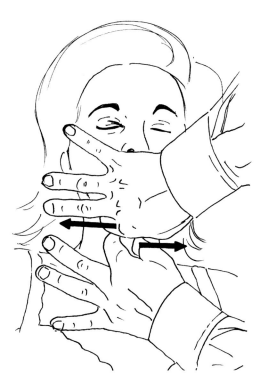

Fig. 8-31 Treatment of the Cervico-Pleural Ligaments

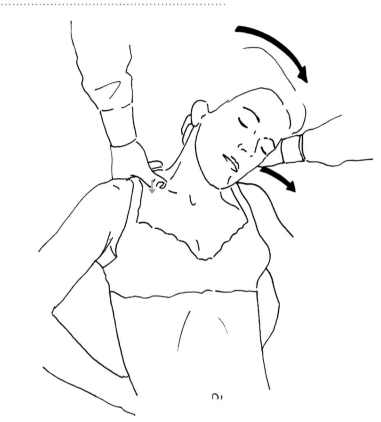

CRANIUM

Scalp

The patient is supine, with the practitioner stationed behind their head. You will find circular areas of slight swellings along with depressed areas around the sutures. Using your finger tip, apply sliding pressure converging towards the center of the restriction (Fig. 8-32). For circular areas, continue into the center and there exert mild pressure, displacing the fascia in all directions with respect to the periosteum (Fig. 8-33).

As previously mentioned, the circular raised areas are often sequelae of shocks and can give rise to lesional chains which propagate downwards. Depressions are usually associated with tiredness, overworking, headaches, and stress.

Occipitocervical junction

The occipitocervical junction is the ultimate area of adaptation and compensation. It is a focus for unremitting tension and it is rare that its movements are completely free.

Fig. 8-32   Treatment of the Exocranial Fasciae: Convergent Pressure

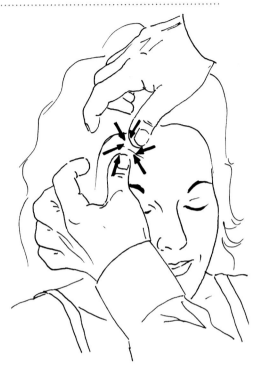

Fig. 8-33   Treatment of the Exocranial Fasciae: Circular Rubbing

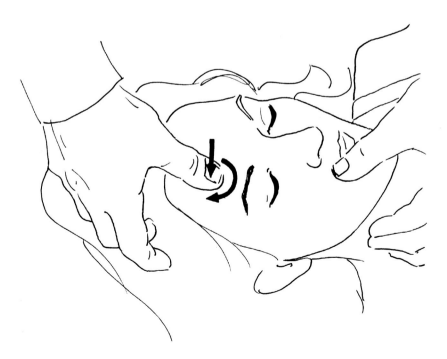

The patient is supine, with the practitioner stationed behind their head. Position the fingers of both hands in the area of soft tissue just below the base of the skull (Fig. 8-34). Exerting mild pressure with the fingers, and monitor the relaxation of the tissues. You can move your hands apart to generate lateral stretching. Finally, at the same time, maintaining the pressure, flex your fingers to generate local stretching in a longitudinal direction.

After this, place the finger tips on the curved line of the occipital ridge. Here, the auricular branch of the vagus nerve passes through an area of osteofibrous tissue and it is not uncommon to find that it is compressed. This is a good opportunity to palpate and then treat a cranial nerve. With just the pressure from the weight of the head, wait for the tissues to relax. If the fingers detect a fascial band or nodular area, treat it accordingly.

Fig. 8-34 Treatment of the Occipitocervical Junction

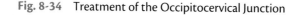

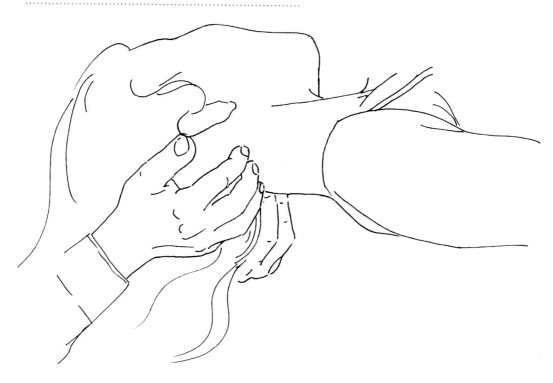

General treatment of the superior fasciae

The patient is supine, with the practitioner stationed behind their head, supporting the base of the skull with both hands in an open V-shape. The thumbs should be placed along the mastoid process and mandible. Generate very mild traction at the same time as readjusting the flexion of the occiput on the atlas to make the traction as specific as possible (Fig. 8-35).

In this position, it is possible to examine all the posterior and lateral fasciae. Depending on the kinds of tension detected, readjust the entire superior segment by small movements of flexion and extension, sidebending, and rotation, and then wait for the tissues to relax. Obviously, if there is a profound disturbance at some remote point, you should specifically treat the problem at its source. The more accurate and specific the treatment, the more likely it is to be effective.

This technique is suitable when the twisting is generalized or as a follow-up procedure to some kind of specific treatment modality. With practice, you will be able to go down quite low in order to complete the technique, but it would be an illusion to think that everything can be treated with this technique.

Fig. 8-35 Global Treatment of the Superior Fasciae

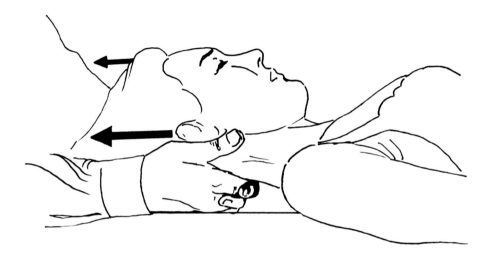

VERTEBRAL DURA MATER

The difference between this technique and the preceding one is very subtle. The patient is supine, with the practitioner stationed behind their head. Both of the practitioner's hands are more or less aligned, one next to the other, along the curved line of the occipital bone. The first step is to readjust the atlas/occiput flexion/extension to align the forces along the axis of the dura mater. Generate very mild traction, more as if you were about to induce such traction rather than actually inducing it. Gradually increase the traction as its effects move down the column (Fig. 8-36).

When you detect a restriction, stop there and, if necessary, adjust sidebending and rotation to focus the forces and wait for the relaxation of the tissues while slightly increasing the tension. Then release the tension and resume it until you feel freedom of movement.

Obviously, if a serious restriction is detected, you must perform a preliminary structural technique rather than hoping for relaxation, which may take an inordinate amount of time. However, for minor tension, or as a complement to a structural technique, this method can be very effective and perfectly suitable.

Fig. 8-36   Treatment of the Vertebral Dura Mater Axis

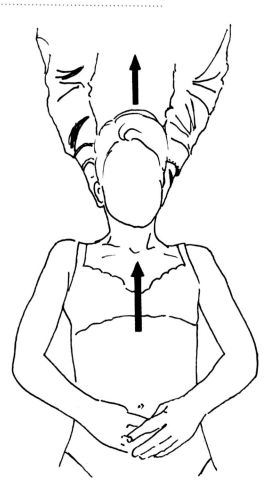

GENERALIZED MANIPULATION OF THE FASCIAE

On the whole, we have been describing local techniques, but relatively generalized or global manipulations of the fasica are also possible, either proceeding region by successive region or addressing an extensive area from the outset. Let us take the lower limb as an example

With the patient supine place one hand on the dorsal surface of the foot and the other in the middle of the tibia. An induction movement will occur between the hands. Harmonize this movement in all spatial planes. Proceed region by successive region up to the hip. Then, with one hand on the foot and the other at the hip, re-harmonize the entire limb (Fig. 8-37). It is also possible to start from the outset at this stage. Starting from the hip, you can move up through the successive regions as far as the cranium.

With a great deal of practice, it is possible to monitor fascial problems from their point of departure, namely, the cranium. Again, this is relevant to generalized tension rather than specific focal points of restriction. It should be recognized that wanting to monitor everything from a single point is extremely ambitious and it may well be wiser to start at the point of the actual restriction, or at least in proximity to it.

Fig. 8-37   Global Treatment of the Fasciae: Lower Limb

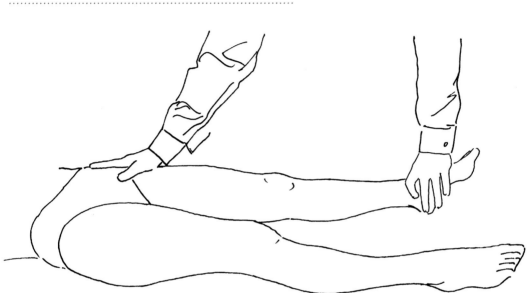

ANTEROPOSTERIOR RE-EQUILIBRATION

This process involves restoring the coordination between the movements of the posterior and anterior fascial elements of the body.

The patient is supine, with the practitioner stationed behind their head, cradling the base of their skull in the left hand. Placing the right hand on the sternum, use the left hand to generate a very mild traction in order to monitor the posterior fasciae (Fig. 8-38). Monitor the anterior fasciae with the right hand, moving along the central axis from the thorax to the epigastrium. By means of listening and induction, harmonize the movements sensed under the hands until complete freedom is obtained and both hands are perfectly synchronized.

STRESS

Many people are permanently in a state of stress, which leaves its mark on the fasciae, disturbing their motility and creating tension, which can further affect their mood. The effect is rather like wearing clothes that are too tight. There is no panacea for this situation and the most suitable treatment strategy will be differ for each person. Nevertheless, osteopathic techniques can help many people, especially if the treatment is undertaken at an early stage.

Fig. 8-38   Anteroposterior Balancing

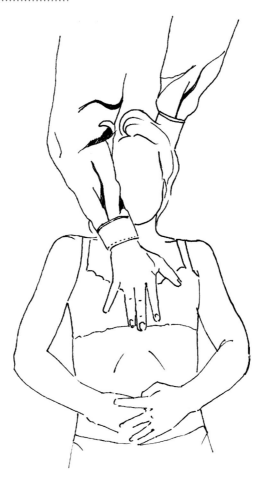

With the patient supine the practitioner takes up a position on either side. Place one hand as flat as possible over the epigastrium. Often you will feel a tense, hard area, as if everything is forming a block, accompanied by abnormally strong aortic pulsations. The tissues will gradually begin to move and relax. It is important for the practitioner to remain perfectly passive and not to try to force the resistant barrier. Ideally, the hand should be able to sink freely into a completely flexible abdomen. Do not forget that the solar plexus lies just below your hand, and that its dysfunction can upset the physiology of the entire area, especially below the transverse mesocolon.

Once this area has relaxed, treat the diaphragm and then continue on to the sternum. Remember that the cardiopulmonary plexus projects to this area, with all the consequences of its dysfunction, which is often related to stress. Finally, turn to the patient's cranium. In each area simply place your hand on the area in question and leave it there until the tissues relax. When you are all done, perform an anteroposterior equilibration and finish with generalized manipulation of the fasciae. Usually this entire process takes 20-30 minutes.

This treatment is not the only possibility—depending on the particular patient, many different variations are possible. However, it has the advantage of conferring a certain degree of well-being which can be long-lasting, particularly if the treatment is undertaken at an early stage in the buildup of stress.

SCARS AND ADHESIONS

It is becoming increasingly rare to encounter a patient with no kind of scar. When a scar becomes a problem, it should be treated without fail because it can represent a primary restriction.

Treat the superficial scar at the level of the scar tissue by longitudinal and transverse stretching. Then continue down to the deeper tissue, because the source of the disturbance is often at this level.

Treatment is performed by identifying the favored axis of motion and then gradually stretching away from the restriction. Come back to the point of departure and stretch again, taking note of the possibilities in the tissues, and gradually including other axes. If necessary, immobilize the fascia on the opposite side of the scar with your other hand. Finish up with listening and induction, which should reveal improved motility of the underlying tissues.

We reiterate that the goal is not to eliminate the adhesions, as this is not really possible. However, irritated adhesions tend to lose elasticity and end up by inhibiting and eventually immobilizing local tissues and organs. For this reason, the goal is to regenerate some degree of elasticity, as this is the potential of all tissues. As a result, the adverse effect of the scar on the organ will be eliminated or significantly attenuated, which will help to preserve its function.

Two common examples are:

- Constipation that commonly follows appendectomy. In some cases, simple manipulation around the postoperative scar can re-establish normal intestinal passage.
- Dyspareunia following an episiotomy, which prevents sexual relations. A single session of treatment of the scar tissue can be sufficient to restore the patient's normal condition.

We could mention many more examples. Not all scars respond well to osteopathic treatment but we believe that it would be wrong to deny patients our potentially beneficial alternative solution.

Treatment Sequence

First of all, it should be emphasized that treatment ought first and foremost to be focused on local problems. It is more elegant, more logical, and more effective to go to the root of the problem in order to correct it. Only later should a generalized correction be considered, such as correction of remote problems transmitted from the primary restriction via a lesional chain. We can then re-equilibrate the entire body around a focal point of restriction which induced the entire, more or less extensive chain reaction.

Re-equilibration of certain fasciae does not necessarily require direct treatment. Listening should be immediately followed by induction, and then rechecked with another listening test.

If direct treatment must be undertaken, begin with listening and induction whenever possible. This will put you in contact with the patient's tissues and establish communication with them. It may also help lower the threshold of irritation as a first step. After this, proceed to direct treatment and then continue by listening and induction, and finally, a listening test.

At the end of the treatment session, it is important to re-test all parameters, including pain and functional mobility. It is important to remember that this will demonstrate to the patient the effectiveness of the osteopathic approach.

Indications and Contraindications

Fascial techniques are non-aggressive and can induce profound changes in the tissues as well as in immune mechanisms and metabolic processes. Given all these benefits, the relevance of these techniques is practically unlimited. It would appear logical that listening and induction can be applied to almost any case.

Contraindications tend to be relative rather than formal. We would advise extreme caution when dealing with infections, and it is not recommended to apply direct techniques on hypersensitive or acutely inflamed tissues.

Direct techniques must never be used on any tension or mass which has not been formally identified as a focus of tissular tension.

As a general rule, one of the over-riding contraindications is never to care for a patient unless you have understood their history and problems. Knowing when to send a patient to someone better equipped to deal with them corresponds to elementary caution and common sense. Even though fascial treatment is relevant to almost all patients, it is not a panacea. It occupies an important position in therapy but should not be accorded more importance than it merits.

Conclusion

When A.T. Still first defined the principles of osteopathy well over a century ago, he emphasized the importance of the fasciae. This is what he said in his *Philosophy of Osteopathy*:

> "I know of no part of the body that equals fascia as a hunting
> ground. I believe that more rich golden thought will appear
> to the mind's eye as the study of the fascia is pursued than
> any division of the body. Still, one part is just as great and
> useful as any other in its place. No part can be dispensed

with. But the fascia is the ground in which all causes of death
do the destruction of life. Every view we take, a wonder
appears."   — *Chapter 1*

"The fascia gives one of, if not the greatest, problems to solve
as to the part it takes in life and death. It belts each muscle,
vein, nerve, and all organs of the body. It is almost a network
of nerves, cells and tubes, running to and from it; it is crossed
and filled with, no doubt, millions of nerve centers and fibers
to carry on the work of secreting and excreting fluid vital and
destructive. By its action we live, and by its failure we shrink,
or swell, and die.   — *Chapter 10*

Every day, new advances in histology and biochemistry confirm Still's intuition. Recent studies have shown that the fasciae play a central role in human physiology. All the various connective tissues in the body can actually be viewed as a single, complex unit which invests specific parenchymatous cells, allowing them to survive and regulating their metabolism. Tissue movements result from constant dynamic interactions among mechanical influences, physiological factors, and their biological consequences.

Advances in research are leading to an ever more profound understanding of the role of tissues, and new results are constantly reinforcing the importance of these roles. New discoveries expand our knowledge and enable us to understand the subtle mechanisms of that marvelous machine, the human body. This improved understanding allows us to develop more effective approaches to correct dysfunction and, as a result, to restore normalcy. This further confirms Still's intuition.

The ubiquity of tissues and the multiplicity of their roles that we have tried to describe leads us to consider restrictions of the fasciae as an integral part of the osteopathic lesion (also known as somatic dysfunction), even as its principal cause. Structure and function are two aspects of a single, indivisible entity. Let us leave the last word to Still:

"There is no real difference between structure and function;
they are just different sides of the same coin. If we learn
nothing about function from the structure, all it means is that
we have not been looking at it in the right way."

Bibliography

Abehsera, A., *Traité de médecine ostéopathique*. Paris: Maloine,1986.

Barone, R., *Anatomie comparée t.2*. Paris: Vigot, 1996.

Barral, J-P., Mercier, P., *Visceral Manipulation*. Seattle: Eastland Press, 1989.

Barral, J-P., Ligner, B., Paoletti, S., Prat, D., Rommeveaux, L., Triana, D. *Nouvelles techniques uro-génitales*. Avignon: Verlaque, 1993.

Bednar, D.A., Orr, F.M., Simon, T., "Observations on the pathomorphology of the thoracolumbar fascia in chronic mechanical back pain." *Spine*: 20(10) 1161-1164, 1995.

Bichat, T.X., *Traité des membranes*. Paris: Mequignon, Marvie, 1816.

Bienfait, M., *Les fascias*. Bordeaux: Ste d'édition médicale—Le Pousoé, 1981.

Blechschmidt, E., *Wie beginnt das menschliche liben vom ei zum embryo*. Stein am Rhein: Christiana-Verlag, 1989.

Boabighi, A., Kuhlmann, J.N., Luboinski, J., Landterit, B., "Aponévroses et fascias superficiels: Propriétés mécaniques et architecturales," *Bull Assoc Anat (Nancy)*. 77(238): 3-7, 1993.

Bouchet, A., Cuillere, T.S., *Anatomie tome 2-4*. Lyon: SIMEAP, 1983.

Bourdinaud, Philippe. *Les techniques tissulaires ostéopathiques péri-articulaires: Tome 1, Le bassin et le traitement général fascia*. Avignon: Verlaque, 2004.

Burger, W., Straube, M., Behne, M., Sarai, K., Beyersdorf, F., Eckel, L., Dereser, A. Satter, P., Kaltenbach, M., "Role of pericardial constraint for right ventricular function in humans." *Chest:* 107 46-49, 1995.

Caporossi, R., Peyralade, F., *Traité pratique d'ostéopathie crânienne.* Avignon: S.I.O. Verlaque, 1993.

Cathie, A.G., "The Fascia of the Body in Relation to Function and Manipulative Therapy." *Academy of Applied Osteopathy Year Book* 1973-1974; 81-84.

Cathie, A.G. "The Influence of the Lower Extremities upon the Structural Integrity of the Body." In Barbara Peterson (Eds.), *Postural Balance and Imbalance.* Indianapolis: American Academy of Osteopathy, 50-53, 1983.

Cisler, T.A., "Whiplash as a total body injury." *JAOA:* 94(2) 145-148, 1994.

Coujard, R., Poirier, J., Racadot, J., *Précis d'Histologie humaine.* Paris: Masson, 1980.

Cruveilher, J., See, M., *Traité d'anatomie descriptive tome* 1, 2, 3. Paris: Asselin, 1877.

Debnar D.A., Orr, T.W., Simon, G.M., "Observation on pathomorphology of the thoracolumbar fascia in chronic mechanical back pain." *Spine:* 20(10) 1163-1664, 1995.

Decramer, M., Jiang T.X., Reid, M.B., Kelly, S., Macklem, P.T., Demedts, M., "Relationship between diaphragm length and abdominal dimensions." *J Appl Physio:* 61(5) 1815-1820, 1986.

Downing, C.H., *Principles and Practice of Osteopathy.* Youngstown, OH: William Publishing Company, 1923.

Drews, U., *Atlas de poche d'embryologie.* Paris: Flammarion, 1994.

Dzubow, L.M., "Tissue movement: A microbiomechanical approach." *J Dermatol Surg—Ancol:* 15 389-399, 1989.

Elias, H., Pauly, J.E., Burns, E.R., *Histologie et microanatomie du corps humain.* Padova: Piccin, 1984.

Erlingheuser, Ralph, F., D.O., "The Circulation of the Cerebrospinal Fluid through the Connective Tissue System." *Academy of Applied Osteopathy Year Book* 1959; 77-87.

Frick, H., Leonhardt, H., Stark, D., *Spezielle anatomie.* Stuttgart: Georg Thieme, 1992.

Frymann, V., *The Collected Papers of Viola M. Frymann, DO: The Legacy of Osteopathy to Children.* Indianapolis, IN: American Academy of Osteopathy, 1998.

Gabarel, B., Roques, M., *Les fascias.* Paris: Maloine, 1994.

Gardner, G., Gray, D.J., Rohull, R.O., *Anatomie.* Paris: Doin, 1979.

Gerlach, H.J., Lierse, W., "Functional construction of the superficial and deep fascia system of the lower limb in man." *Acta Anat*: 139 11-25, 1990.

Gregoire, R., Oberlin, S., *Précis d'anatomie*. Paris: J.B. Baillere, 1948.

Hack, G.D., Koritzer, R.T., Robinson, W.L., Hallgren, R.C., Greenman, P.E. "Anatomic relation between the rectus capitis posterior minor muscle and the dura mater." *Spine*: 20(23) 2484-2486, 1995.

Haegel, P., Moore, K., *Eléments d'embryologie humaine*. Paris: Vigot, 1995.

Harisson, T.R., *Principes de médecine interne*. Paris: Flammarion, 1975.

Hohne, K.H., Pelesser, B., Pommert, A., Riemer, M., Schielmann, T.H., Schubert, R., Tiede, U., "A New representation of knowledge concerning human anatomy and function." *Nature Medicine*: 1 (6) 506-511, 1995.

Huidobro-Toro, J.P., Harris, R.A., "Brain lipids that induce sleep are novel modulators of 5-hydroxytryptamine receptors." *Proc Natl Acad Sci*: 93 8078-8082, July 1996.

Hurschler, C., Vanderby Jr., R., Martinez, D.A., Vialas, A.G., Turnispeed, W.D., "Mechanical and biomechanical analyses of tibial compartment fascia in chronic compartment syndrome." *An of Biomech Eng*: 22 272-279, 1994.

Issartel, L., Issartel, M., *L'ostéopathie exactement*. Paris: Laffont, 1983.

Jones, L.H., *Correction spontanée par positionnement*. Charleroi: OMC, 1995.

Junqueira, L.C., Carneiro, J., *Histologie*. Padova: Piccin, 1982.

Kahle, W., Leonhardt, H., Platzer, W., *Anatomie—tome* 1, 2, 3. Paris: Flammarion, 1979.

Kahn, M.F., Peltier, A., *Maladies sytémiques*. Paris: Flammarion, 1982.

Kamina, P., *Petit bassin et périnée*. Paris: Maloine, 1998.

Kamina, P., *Abdomen*. Paris: Maloine, 1998.

Kamina, P., *Anatomie générale*. Paris: Maloine, 1996.

Korr, I.M., *Bases physiologiques de l'ostéopathie*. Bruxelles: SBO RTM, 1982.

Krassimira, N.M., "Development of the human fetal visceral pleura: An ultra structural study." *Ann Anat*: 178 91-99, 1996.

Kuchiwaki, H., Suguru, I., Nahohiro, I., Yukio, O., Nobumitsu, S., "Changes in dural thickness reflect changes in intracranial pressure in dogs." *Neuroscience Letters*: 198(1) 68-70, Sep 22, 1995.

Kühne, L.W., *Atlas de poche d'histologie*. Paris: Flammarion, 1986.

Langman, J., *Embryologie humaine*. Paris: Masson, 1976.

Lazorthes, G., *Le système nerveux central*. Paris: Masson, 1986.

Lazorthes, G., *Le système nerveux périphérique*. Paris: Masson, 1981.

Lewitt, K. "The needle effect in relief of myofascial pain." *Pain*: 6, 83-90, 1979.

Magoun, H.J., "Fascia in the Writings of A.T. Still." *J Osteopath Cranial Assoc*, Meridian, Idaho: The Cranial Academy, 47, 1954.

Magoun, H.J., *Osteopathy in the Cranial Field*. 3rd ed. Kirksville: Journal Printing Company, 1976.

Melzack, R., Wall, P.O., *Le défi de la douleur*. Paris: Maloine, 1982.

Nusslein-Volhard, C., "Gradients that organize embryo development." *Scientific American*: 297 (August 1996): 54-61.

Nicholas, D.S., Weller, R.O., "The fine anatomy of the human spinal meninges." *J of Neurosurg*: 69 276-282, 1988.

Page, L.E., "The Role of the Fascae in the Maintenance of Structural Integrity." *Academy of Applied Osteopathy Year Book* 1952; 70-73.

Paiva, M., Verbanck, S., Estenne, M., Poncelet, B., Segebarth, C., Macklem, P.T., "Mechanical implications of in vivo human diaphragm shape." *J Appl Physio*: 72(4):1407-1412, 1992.

Palastanga, N., Field, D., Samoes, R., *Anatomy in Human Function*. Oxford: Butterworth-Heinemann, 1991.

Parkinson, D., "Human spinal arachnoid septa, trabeculae, and 'rogue strands'." *Am J of Anat*: 192 498-509, 1991.

Pequignot, H., *Pathologie médicale*. Paris: Masson, 1979.

Pischinger, A., *Matrix & Matrix Regulation: Basis for a Holistic Theory in Medicine*. Portland, OR: Medicina Biologica, 1991.

Pillet, J., *Anatomie du petit bassin*. Paris: Doin, 1978.

Poirier, J., Ribadeau Dumas., J.L., *Histologie*. Paris: Masson, 1995.

Poirier, J., Cohen, I., Baudet, J., *Embryologie humaine*. Paris: Maloine, 1996.

Rolf, I.P. *Rolfing: The Integration of Human Structures*. New York: Harper Collins Publishers, 1978.

Rouviere, H., Delmas, A., *Anatomie – tome 1, 2, 3.* Paris: Masson, 1959.

Rydevik, B., Holm, S., Brown, M.D., Lunborg, G., "Diffusion from the cerebrospinal fluid as a nutritional pathway for spinal nerve roots." *Acta Physio Scandinavia:* 138 (2) 247-248, 1990.

Signoret, J., Collenot, R., *L'organisme en développement.* Paris: Hermann, 1996.

Snyder, G.E., "Fasciae: Applied Anatomy and Physiology." *Academy of Applied Osteopathy Year Book* 1956; 65-75.

Stevens, A., Lowe, J.S., *Histologie.* Paris: Pradel, 1996.

Stevenson S., Cunningham N., Toth J., Davy D., Reddi A.H., "The effect of osteogenin (a bone morphogenetic protein) on the formation of bone in orthotopic segmental defects in rats." *J Bone Joint Surg Am* 76:1676-87, 1994.

Still, A.T., *Osteopathy: Research and Practice.* Seattle: Eastland Press, Reprint 1992.

Stryer, L., *Biochimie.* Paris: Flammarion, 1988.

Testut, L., *Traité d'anatomie humaine.* Paris: O. Doin, 1891.

Tuchmann Duplessis, H., *Embryologie.* Paris: Masson, 1974.

Toldt, C., *Anotomis her atlas.* Vienne: Urban et Schwarzenberg, 1894.

Typaldos, S., "Introducing the fascial distortion model." *AAO Journal* 4:2: 14-18, 30-36, 1994.

Typaldos, S., "Triggerband technique." *AAO Journal* 4:4: 15-18, 30-33, 1994.

Typaldos, S., "Continuum technique." *AAO Journal* 5:2: 15-19, 1995.

Upledger, J.E., Vredevoogd, J., *Craniosacral Therapy.* Chicago: Eastland Press, 1983.

Upledger, J.E., *Craniosacral Therapy II: Beyond the Dura.* Seattle: Eastland Press, 1987.

Verschakelen, J.A., Deschepper, K., Jiang, J.X., Demedts, M., "Diaphragmatic displacement measured by fluroroscopy and derived by respitrace." *J Appl Physio:* 67(2): 694-698, 1989.

Vleeming, A, Pool-Goudzwaard, A.L., Stoeckart, R., van Wingerden J.P., Snijders C.J., "The posterior layer of the thoracolumbar fascia: Its function in load transfer from spine to legs." *Spine:* 20(7) 753-758, 1995.

Waligora, J., Perlemuter, L., *Anatomie abdomen et petit bassin.* Paris: Masson, 1974.

Weil, J.H., *Biochimie générale*. Paris: Masson, 1997.

Wright, S., *Physiologie appliquée à la médecine*. Paris: Flammarion, 1984.

Yahia, L.H., Pigeon, P., Desrosiers, E.A., "Viscoelastic properties of the human lumbodorsal fascia." *J Biomed Eng*: 5 425-429, 1993.

Yahia, L.H., Rhalmi, S., Newman, N., Isler, M., "Sensory innervation of human thoraco-lumbar fascia." *Acta Orthop Scandinavia*: 63 (2) 195-197, 1992.

Yaszemski, M.J., Augustus, M., "The discectomy membrane (nerve root fibrovascular membrane): Its anatomic description and its surgical importance." *J Spinal Dis*: 7 (3) 230-235, 1994.

Index

Bold page numbers indicate that the item appears in an illustration.

M